Advances in Pleural Diseases - Molecular and Surgical Perspectives

Edited by Güntuğ Batıhan

Published in London, United Kingdom

Advances in Pleural Diseases - Molecular and Surgical Perspectives
http://dx.doi.org/10.5772/intechopen.1008662
Edited by Güntuğ Batıhan

Contributors
Basil Younis, Berivan Karatekin Usta, Fatma Selen Ala Çitlak, Güntuğ Batıhan, Hsin-Yi Wang, İlker Kolbaş, Jin-Yuan Shih, Maricar Rulloda-Agoncillo, Mohammad Alabdallat, Richard L. Kradin, Ömer Faruk Sağlam, Ömer Selim Unat

First published in London, United Kingdom, 2026 by IntechOpen
IntechOpen is the global imprint of INTECHOPEN LIMITED, registered in England and Wales, registration number: 11086078, 167-169 Great Portland Street, London, W1W 5PF, United Kingdom

For EU product safety concerns: IN TECH d.o.o., Prolaz Marije Krucifikse Kozulić 3, 51000 Rijeka, Croatia, info@intechopen.com or visit our website at intechopen.com.

British Library Cataloguing-in-Publication Data
A catalogue record for this book is available from the British Library

Advances in Pleural Diseases - Molecular and Surgical Perspectives
Edited by Güntuğ Batıhan
p. cm.
Print ISBN 978-1-83635-157-3
Online ISBN 978-1-83635-156-6
eBook (PDF) ISBN 978-1-83635-158-0

If disposing of this product, please recycle the paper responsibly.

Meet the editor

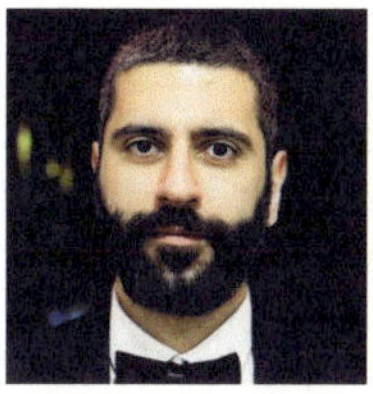

Dr. Güntuğ Batıhan is an Associate Professor of Thoracic Surgery at Çanakkale Onsekiz Mart University. He specializes in minimally invasive thoracic surgery, particularly video-assisted thoracoscopic surgery (VATS), complex anatomical lung resections, airway surgery, and pleural diseases. His academic work focuses on thoracic surgery, clinical investigation, and the continuous refinement of surgical techniques through research and innovation. Dr. Batıhan has authored numerous peer-reviewed publications and book chapters and actively contributes to international scientific collaborations. He serves in editorial roles for international journals and is an active member of several international thoracic and respiratory societies. He is involved in surgical education, academic publishing, and multidisciplinary thoracic care. He is committed to advancing thoracic surgery through scientific rigor, innovation, and the integration of emerging technologies into clinical practice.

Contents

Preface

Pleural diseases occupy a distinctive and increasingly significant position within thoracic medicine and surgery. Situated at the interface between lung parenchyma and chest wall, the pleura reflects a broad spectrum of physiological, inflammatory, infectious, environmental, and malignant processes. In recent decades, the field has evolved from a largely descriptive discipline into one shaped by advances in molecular diagnostics, biomarker research, imaging technologies, and minimally invasive surgical techniques.

This book has been conceived to present pleural disease as an integrated field rather than a collection of isolated conditions. It brings together foundational concepts in pleural anatomy and pathophysiology with contemporary diagnostic strategies, including radiologic assessment and molecular analysis. At the same time, it addresses the clinical management of both benign and malignant pleural disorders, emphasizing the growing role of minimally invasive thoracic surgery.

Throughout the volume, attention is given not only to traditional clinical entities such as pleural thickening and empyema, but also to emerging areas including biomarker-driven diagnostics and pleural fluid–based molecular testing in lung cancer. The integration of biological insight with clinical application reflects the broader transformation of thoracic medicine toward precision and individualized care.

Surgical management is discussed within the context of technological innovation, particularly the expansion of video-assisted thoracoscopic techniques. The shift toward less invasive approaches represents a defining feature of modern pleural intervention and underscores the importance of combining sound biological understanding with refined operative strategy.

Taken together, the chapters aim to provide a balanced and contemporary overview of pleural diseases, bridging basic science, translational research, and clinical practice. By approaching pleural pathology from multiple complementary perspectives, this book seeks to contribute to a more coherent, biologically informed understanding of the field.

I would like to express my sincere gratitude to all contributing authors for their scholarly expertise, dedication, and collaborative spirit. Their work has shaped this book into a comprehensive and multidisciplinary resource. I am also grateful to the publishing team for their professional guidance and support throughout the editorial process.

I hope this volume will serve as a valuable reference for clinicians, surgeons, researchers, and trainees seeking a deeper, more integrated understanding of pleural disease in contemporary thoracic practice.

Güntuğ Batıhan
Department of Thoracic Surgery,
Canakkale Onsekiz Mart University,
Canakkale, Turkey

Section 1

Fundamentals of Pleural Biology

Chapter 1

Pleural Diseases: Anatomy, Physiology, and Pathophysiology

Ömer Selim Unat

Abstract

The pleura is a double-layered serous membrane that envelops the lungs and lines the thoracic cavity, playing a pivotal role in respiratory mechanics and host defense. This chapter reviews the pleural anatomy, histology, physiology, and pathophysiology, providing a foundational understanding of pleural structure and function. The visceral pleura, derived from splanchnic mesoderm, closely adheres to the lung parenchyma and is innervated by autonomic fibers, while the parietal pleura, of somatic origin, lines the thoracic wall and has rich somatic innervation. The pleural cavity contains a small volume of lubricating fluid, maintained by a balance between hydrostatic and oncotic pressures and efficient lymphatic drainage. Disruption of this balance may lead to pleural effusion or pneumothorax. Furthermore, chronic inflammation can result in pleural thickening, impairing respiratory mechanics. Understanding pleural physiology, particularly fluid dynamics and pressure regulation, is essential for interpreting pleural pathologies and guiding interventions such as thoracentesis. Special emphasis is given to Starling forces, mesothelial cell function, and the role of manometry in assessing pleural elastance. This integrated overview supports the clinical and diagnostic approach to pleural diseases.

Keywords: pleura, pleural fluid dynamics, pleural effusion, visceral and parietal pleura, pleura anatomy

1. Introduction

The pleura, as an essential component of the respiratory system, plays a critical role not only in facilitating lung mechanics but also in host defense, fluid regulation, and response to injury. Structurally, it is a double-layered membrane that completely surrounds the lungs, forming a barrier between the lung surface and the thoracic wall. The inner layer covering the lung surface is called the visceral pleura, while the outer layer adjacent to the thoracic wall is known as the parietal pleura. Together, these layers enclose a potential space – the pleural cavity – which normally contains a small amount of pleural fluid (**Figure 1**) [1].

The pleural membranes and the pleural cavity facilitate smooth lung movement within the thoracic cavity – particularly during deep or heavy breathing – by

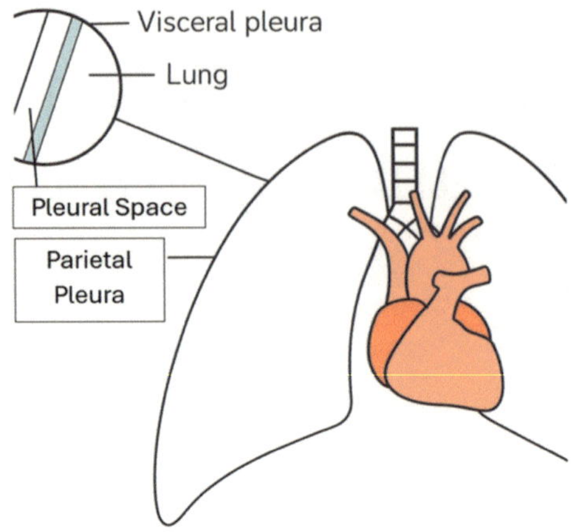

Figure 1.
Diagram of the pleural space.

reducing friction and serving as a protective barrier between the lungs and surrounding structures [2].

Diseases of the pleura can lead to the accumulation of air, fluid, or blood in the potential space of the pleural cavity, or to the impairment of the pleura's lubricating function, which normally facilitates respiration. These disorders may originate from the pleura itself or result from systemic diseases. In this chapter, we will discuss the anatomy, physiology, and pathophysiology of the pleura to provide a foundation for understanding pleural diseases.

2. Anatomy and histology of pleura

2.1 Visceral pleura

The visceral pleura completely envelops the lung parenchyma and is composed of a single layer of cuboidal mesothelial cells. Beneath this mesothelial layer lie a basement membrane and submesothelial connective tissue [3]. Embryologically, the visceral pleura originates from the splanchnic mesoderm, while the parietal pleura arises from the somatic (parietal) mesoderm [4]. Due to their distinct embryological origins, the visceral and parietal pleurae have different vascular supplies.

As the visceral pleura completely envelops the lungs, it also extends into and covers the fissures between the lobes. In the right lung, it lines both the major (oblique) and minor (horizontal) fissures, while in the left lung, it covers the major fissure. In cases of pleural effusion, fluid may occasionally accumulate within the interlobar fissures, mimicking parenchymal lesions on imaging studies (**Figure 2**) [5].

The lymphatic drainage of the visceral pleura is directed inward into the lung parenchyma, where it forms dense plexuses that converge at the hilum and drain into the bronchial lymphatic vessels [6].

DOI: http://dx.doi.org/10.5772/intechopen.1012438

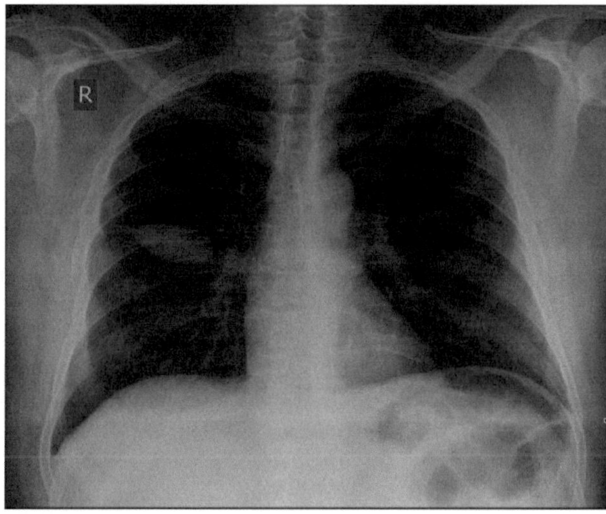

Figure 2.
Lung pseudotumor caused by fluid accumulation in fissure. (Image source: Radiopaedia.org, Case r-19942. Licensed under CC BY–NC–SA 3.0.).

2.2 Parietal pleura

The parietal pleura is in close anatomical relationship with thoracic and mediastinal structures. Based on the regions it contacts within the thoracic cavity, it is divided into four parts [2]:

1) Cervical pleura: It covers the apex of the lung and the inner surface of the thoracic inlet above the first rib.

2) Costal pleura: It lines the inner surface of the ribs and the intercostal spaces.

3) Diaphragmatic pleura: It covers the superior surface of the diaphragm.

4) Mediastinal pleura: It lies adjacent to the mediastinum and covers its lateral aspect.

The cervical pleura lines the inner surface of the thoracic inlet bilaterally. Several vital structures pass through the thoracic inlet, including the brachiocephalic arteries and veins, branches of the brachial plexus, the vagus nerve, the esophagus, and the trachea. The thoracic cavity is divided by the mediastinum, and the mediastinal pleura lies in close proximity to the heart, great vessels, and the pericardium that encloses them [2].

Between the mediastinal and costal pleura, there is a narrow pleural space known as the costomediastinal recess, located in the anterior thorax. This recess is typically more prominent on the left side, where the anterolateral portion of the left lower lobe may expand into it during inspiration. Because of this dynamic movement, the costomediastinal recess is clinically significant, as pleural fluid may accumulate in this area in cases of pleural effusion [6]. A cross-sectional diagram of the thorax depicting pleural structures is shown in **Figure 3**.

A pleural recess, known as the costophrenic recess, is located between the costal and diaphragmatic pleura. One of the earliest radiographic signs of pleural effusion is the blunting of the costophrenic angles, which reflects fluid accumulation in this space (**Figure 4**) [6].

At the level of the upper mediastinum, the right and left parietal pleurae come into close contact posterior to the sternum. Under normal conditions, there is little-to-no space between these pleural reflections. However, when lung volume decreases – such as during expiration, in restrictive lung diseases, or in cases of lung collapse – this potential space may expand, creating a noticeable separation between the pleural layers. This phenomenon is more pronounced in infants, thin individuals, or during deep expiration, and may be visible radiographically as a lucent area in the anterior mediastinum [7].

The parietal pleura receives its arterial blood supply primarily from the intercostal arteries, whereas the mediastinal portion is supplied by the superior phrenic and musculophrenic arteries. Venous drainage of the parietal pleura occurs through the intercostal veins. In contrast, the visceral pleura is supplied by the bronchial arteries and drains via the pulmonary veins, highlighting a key difference in vascularization between the two pleural layers [8].

The parietal pleura possesses a rich and well-organized lymphatic network, which plays a critical role in the absorption of pleural fluid and the clearance of cellular debris or pathogens from the pleural space. Lymphatic vessels are particularly dense in the costal, mediastinal, and diaphragmatic regions. These vessels drain into the intercostal, parasternal, mediastinal, and diaphragmatic lymph nodes, depending on the specific pleural surface. Unlike the visceral pleura, which drains into intrapulmonary nodes, the parietal pleura drains externally, making it a primary route for pleural fluid resorption [9].

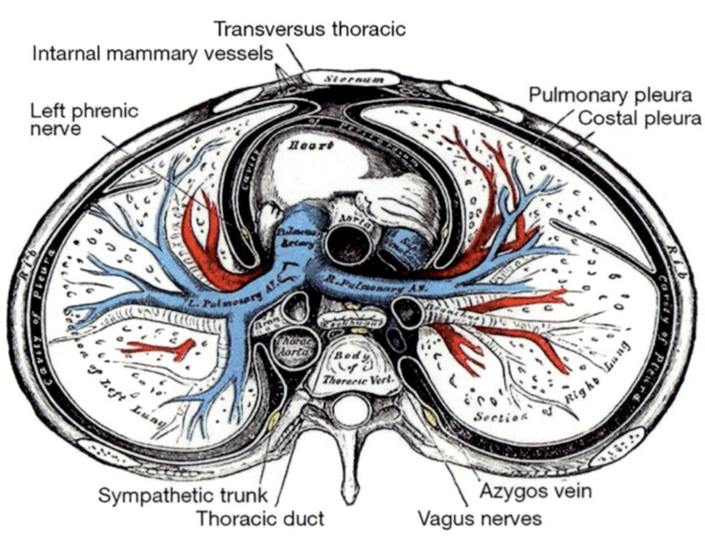

Figure 3.
Schematic cross-section of the thorax illustrating the pleural space.

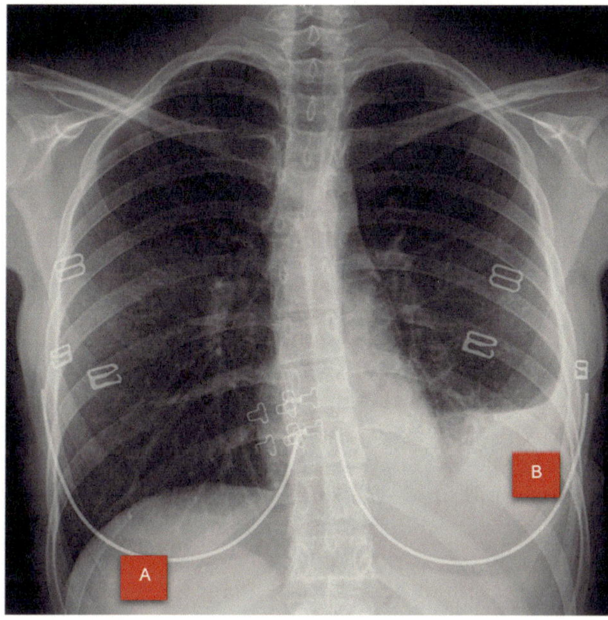

Figure 4.
Left-sided pleural effusion with loss of the costophrenic angle: a) The right costophrenic sinus is clearly visible. b) On the left, the costophrenic angle is obscured due to pleural effusion. Additionally, a damoiseau line is visible, indicating fluid accumulation (Image from the author's own archive).

2.3 Innervation of pleura

The innervation of the pleura differs significantly between its two layers and has important clinical implications. The visceral pleura is innervated by the autonomic nervous system, specifically by vagal and sympathetic nerve fibers that accompany the bronchovascular structures. These fibers primarily regulate vasomotor tone and are not sensitive to somatic pain. As a result, pathological processes involving the visceral pleura, such as early-stage pleural effusion or tumor infiltration, typically do not produce pain unless the parietal pleura or adjacent somatic structures are affected [6, 10].

In contrast, the parietal pleura receives rich somatic innervation, rendering it extremely sensitive to pain, touch, and temperature. The costal pleura and peripheral portion of the diaphragmatic pleura are supplied by the intercostal nerves, whereas the mediastinal pleura and central diaphragmatic pleura are innervated by the phrenic nerve (C3–C5) [6, 11]. Irritation or inflammation of the parietal pleura, such as in pleuritis or pneumothorax, causes sharp and localized chest pain that typically worsens with respiration or coughing. Involvement of the phrenic nerve may also result in referred pain to the shoulder or neck, providing a useful clinical clue for the location of pleural pathology [11].

2.4 Histology of pleura

On the surface facing the pleural cavity, the parietal pleura is lined by a single layer of mesothelial cells, beneath which lies connective tissue adjacent to the thoracic wall and vasculature. This submesothelial connective tissue contains capillaries and lymphatic lacunae, which are integral to pleural fluid drainage. The lacunae are connected to the pleural space via mesothelial stomata, forming a direct interface between the pleural cavity and the lymphatic system. The thickness of the parietal pleura is approximately 20–25 μm, while the underlying connective tissue of the thoracic wall measures around 100–150 μm [6, 8].

The pleural submesothelial layer contains matrix proteins such as fibronectin, which support tissue integrity and mesothelial repair. Mesothelial cells also produce hyaluronic acid, aiding lubrication and immune modulation. Inflammation alters these components: Fibronectin and vitronectin increase, while fragmented hyaluronic acid may promote fibrosis and effusion [12].

In clinical practice, during procedures such as thoracentesis or chest tube insertion in patients with pleural effusion or pneumothorax, the physician must traverse the skin, subcutaneous tissue, and thoracic wall to reach the parietal pleura. The goal is to access the pleural space – the potential area between the parietal and visceral pleura – where fluid or air has accumulated. Minor bleeding may occur due to disruption of subpleural capillaries, and pain may be elicited due to the rich somatic innervation of the parietal pleura.

In contrast, the visceral pleura consists of a single layer of mesothelial cells containing numerous microvilli. These structures not only increase the surface area to support pleural fluid resorption but also contribute to lubrication by producing hyaluronic acid-rich glycoproteins, thereby facilitating frictionless lung movement [6, 8, 13].

3. Physiology of pleura

At the end of expiration, when the lungs reach functional residual capacity, the pleural pressure typically falls to approximately –6 cm H_2O. This negative pleural pressure results from the elastic recoil of the lungs opposing the expansive tendency of the chest wall. During inspiration, the descent of the diaphragm and expansion of the thoracic cavity further increase the negativity of pleural pressure [14].

During expiration, especially during forced expiration, pleural pressure remains negative but may approach positive values. This consistently negative pressure plays a critical role in facilitating inspiration [15].

Additionally, the presence of a glycoprotein-rich fluid between the mesothelial layers of the pleura allows the pleural surfaces to slide smoothly over one another, thereby reducing friction and facilitating efficient respiratory mechanics [15].

Under physiological conditions, the pleural space contains approximately 5–15 mL of fluid [6]. This fluid plays a crucial role in lubricating the visceral and parietal pleurae, allowing frictionless movement during respiration. On average, around 15–20 mL of pleural fluid is produced per day, mostly from the systemic capillaries of the parietal pleura, and an equivalent amount is absorbed via lymphatics to maintain homeostasis [14].

Pleural fluid is a clear, pale yellow ultrafiltrate of plasma with low protein and LDH concentrations. Its cellular content is typically low, with a predominance of macrophages (~75%), followed by lymphocytes (~23%), and a small number of mesothelial cells (~1%) [16]. These mesothelial cells line both pleural surfaces and play active roles in immune modulation and fluid dynamics.

Importantly, mesothelial cells are fragile and can detach easily from the pleural surface, especially during disease states or even minimal mechanical irritation. This can lead to underrepresentation in cytological specimens and must be considered during fluid analysis [17].

Pleural fluid volume is tightly regulated by the equilibrium between hydrostatic and oncotic forces across pleural capillaries and efficient lymphatic drainage. Filtration is driven by hydrostatic pressure gradients – particularly from parietal pleural capillaries into the pleural space – while oncotic pressure opposes this movement. Under physiological conditions, pleural fluid is produced at a rate of approximately 0.15 mL/kg/hour, totaling about 250 mL/day in an average adult. The lymphatic system has a remarkably high resorptive capacity – capable of absorbing up to 28 times the daily fluid production, equating to a theoretical maximum of 7,000 mL/day. This dynamic balance ensures minimal fluid accumulation in the pleural space under normal conditions. Mesothelial cells actively participate in both the production and clearance of pleural fluid. Disruption in this balance – due to elevated hydrostatic pressure (e.g., in heart failure) or decreased oncotic pressure – leads to transudative effusions, while inflammatory or structural pleural damage causes exudates. Cardiopulmonary cyclic pressures further modulate pleural pressure fluctuations, subtly affecting fluid dynamics and venous return efficiency [18].

Monitoring pleural pressure during thoracentesis using pleural manometry provides insights into pleural elastance – it is defined as the change in pleural pressure relative to the volume of fluid removed. Light et al. described three characteristic elastance curves: normal, entrapped, and trapped lung [19]. In a trapped lung, due to chronic inflammation and a fibrous visceral peel, the pleural pressure may already be negative before drainage begins and falls steeply during the procedure, often accompanied by high pleural elastance (>25 cm H_2O/L). In contrast, an entrapped lung – associated with active inflammation or endobronchial obstruction – displays a biphasic pressure–volume curve and is frequently symptomatic. Manometry can also help prevent complications such as re-expansion pulmonary edema, pneumothorax, and chest pain by guiding early termination of thoracentesis when pressures fall below thresholds such as –20 cm H_2O (**Table 1**) [20, 21].

4. Pleural pathophysiology

The pleural space plays a vital role in respiration by maintaining a negative pleural pressure relative to atmospheric pressure. This negative pressure ensures that the lungs remain expanded within the thoracic cavity. The difference between alveolar pressure and pleural pressure is referred to as the transpulmonary pressure. This pressure gradient is crucial for lung inflation: during inspiration, diaphragm contraction and chest wall expansion further decrease the pleural pressure, increasing the transpulmonary pressure and allowing air to enter the lungs [6, 22]. Any disturbance in this pressure relationship can result in impaired ventilation and gas exchange.

Component	Normal values
Total volume	5–15 mL
Daily production	15–20 mL/day
Appearance	Clear, pale yellow
Protein	<1.5 g/dL
LDH	<50% of serum
Cellularity	700–3,000 cells/mL
Main cell types	Macrophages (~75%), lymphocytes (~23%), mesothelial cells (~1%)

Table 1 *was generated based on data from Refs. [20, 21].*

Table 1.
Normal pleural fluid characteristics.

4.1 Pneumothorax and pleural pressure increase

In pneumothorax, air enters the pleural space, leading to a rise in pleural pressure toward atmospheric or even positive values. This eliminates the normal negative pressure gradient, causing lung collapse due to the unopposed elastic recoil of the lung [23]. The resulting hypoxemia is primarily due to ventilation-perfusion mismatch and shunt physiology.

In tension pneumothorax, the condition becomes life-threatening as the pleural pressure exceeds atmospheric pressure with each breath, leading to progressive compression of the ipsilateral lung, contralateral mediastinal shift, and compression of the great vessels. This results in reduced venous return to the heart, hypotension, and possible cardiovascular collapse [24].

4.2 Mechanisms of pleural effusion formation

Pleural effusion results from an imbalance in fluid production and absorption in the pleural space. The major pathophysiologic mechanisms include the following:

1. Increased hydrostatic pressure: Seen in congestive heart failure, elevated pressure in the systemic or pulmonary circulation promotes fluid movement into the pleural space [25].

2. Increased vascular permeability: Inflammatory states (e.g., pneumonia, malignancy) disrupt endothelial integrity, allowing protein-rich fluid to leak into the pleural space [26].

3. Decreased oncotic pressure: Conditions such as nephrotic syndrome or cirrhosis lower plasma oncotic pressure, reducing the reabsorption of fluid from the pleural space [27].

4. Atelectasis-associated effusion: Collapse of lung parenchyma creates increased negative intrapleural pressure, favoring fluid accumulation [28].

5. Impaired lymphatic drainage: As seen in chylothorax, where thoracic duct obstruction or trauma leads to the accumulation of lipid-rich lymph in the pleural space [29].

4.3 Pleural thickening and respiratory impairment

Chronic inflammation or injury to the pleura may lead to pleural thickening, which can restrict lung expansion and impair respiratory mechanics. Patients may present with dyspnea and a restrictive pattern on pulmonary function testing. Common causes include the following:

- Previous tuberculous pleuritis
- Residual fibrosis post-empyema
- Asbestos-related pleural plaques, typically due to occupational or environmental exposure [30, 31].

Pleural thickening may reduce thoracic compliance, increase the work of breathing, and contribute to chronic respiratory insufficiency in severe cases.

5. Conclusion(s)

The pleura is fundamental to efficient respiration, acting as a dynamic interface between the lungs and the thoracic cavity. The parietal pleura lines the thoracic wall and forms anatomical recesses such as the costophrenic and costomediastinal sinuses, which are clinically significant sites for fluid accumulation. Owing to its rich somatic innervation, the parietal pleura is highly sensitive to pain, making pleural irritation or inflammation symptomatic. In contrast, the visceral pleura completely envelops the lung parenchyma and, due to its autonomic innervation, is relatively insensitive to pain. Understanding these anatomical and physiological distinctions is essential for interpreting pleural pathology, such as effusion or thickening, which disrupts normal pleural dynamics and impairs respiratory function. A comprehensive knowledge of pleural structure, innervation, and fluid regulation provides a critical foundation for the diagnosis and management of pleural diseases.

Conflict of interest

The author reports no funding sources and no competing interests in connection with this work.

Author details

Ömer Selim Unat[1,2]

1 Health Sciences University, Izmir Dr. Suat Sern Chest Diseases and Surgery Training and Research Hospital, Pulmonology Department, Izmir, Türkiye

2 Ege University, Health Sciences Institute, Izmir, Türkiye

*Address all correspondence to: unatomerselim@gmail.com

References

[1] Lee KF, Olak J. Anatomy and physiology of the pleural space. Chest Surgery Clinics of North America. 1994;**4**:391–403

[2] Charalampidis C, Youroukou A, Lazaridis G, Baka S, Mpoukovinas I, Karavasilis V, et al. Pleura space anatomy. Journal of Thoracic Disease. 2015;**7**(S1):S27–32. DOI: 10.3978/j.issn.2072-1439.2015.01.48

[3] Adeyinka A, Pierre L. Air Leak. In: StatPearls [Internet]. StatPearls Publishing: Treasure Island (FL); 2023

[4] Durland JL, Sferlazzo M, Logan M, Burke AC. Visualizing the lateral somitic frontier in the Prx1Cre transgenic mouse. Journal of Anatomy. 2008;**212**:590–602. 10.1111/j.1469-7580.2008.00879.x

[5] Fraser RS, Müller NL, Colman N, Paré PD. English, Book, USA, 9780721661940, (Ed.4), Philadelphia, Fraser and Paré's diagnosis of diseases of the chest. Philadelphia, Pennsylvania, USA: W.B. Saunders; 1999. vols. **1-4**:xlii+3190

[6] Light RW. Pleural Diseases. 6th ed. Philadelphia: Lippincott Williams & Wilkins; 2013

[7] Standring S, editor. Gray's Anatomy: The Anatomical Basis of Clinical Practice. 42nd ed. New York: Elsevier; 2020. p. 958–961

[8] Yılmaz N.Plevranın anatomisi ve histolojisi. Solunum. 2002;**4**(Suppl 1):73–75

[9] Gaudio E, Rendina EA, Pannarale L, Ricci C, Marinozzi G. Surface morphology of the human pleura: A scanning electron microscopic study. Chest, Volume. 1988;**93**(1):149–153

[10] Hough A. Physiotherapy in Respiratory Care: An Evidence-Based Approach to Respiratory and Cardiac Management. 3rd ed. Cheltenham, UK: Nelson Thornes; 2001

[11] Agostoni E, Zocchi L. Mechanical coupling and pleural space innervation. In: Geffroy Y, editor. The Pleura in Health and Disease. Boca Raton (FL), USA: CRC Press; 2003. p. 123–134

[12] Mutsaers SE. 2004. The mesothelial cell. The International Journal of Biochemistry & Cell Biology. **36**(1): 9–16. DOI: 10.1016/s1357-2725(03)00242-5

[13] Batra H, Antony VB. 2015. Pleural mesothelial cells in pleural and lung diseases. Journal of Thoracic Disease. 7(6):964–980. DOI: 10.3978/j.issn.2072-1439.2015.02.19

[14] Agostoni E. 1972. Mechanics of the pleural space. Physiological Reviews. **52**(1):57–128. DOI: 10.1152/physrev.1972.52.1.57

[15] DeBiasi EM, Feller-Kopman D. 2021. Anatomy and applied physiology of the pleural space. Clinics in Chest Medicine. **42**(4):567–576. DOI: 10.1016/j.ccm.2021.08.005

[16] Noppen M, De Waele M, Li R, et al. Volume and cellular content of normal pleural fluid in humans examined by pleural lavage. American Journal of Respiratory and Critical Care Medicine. 2000;**162**: 1023–1026

[17] Antony VB, Sahn SA. Pleural biology in health and disease. The American review of respiratory disease. 1993;**147**(6 Pt 1):1635–1656. DOI: 10.1164/ajrccm/147.6_Pt_1.1635

[18] Ferreiro L, Toubes ME, Suárez-Antelo J, Rodríguez-Núñez N, Valdés L. Clinical overview of the physiology and pathophysiology of pleural fluid movement: A narrative review. ERJ Open Research. 2024;**10**(5): 00050–2024. DOI: 10.1183/23120541.00050-2024

[19] Light RW, Jenkinson SG, Minh VD, George RB. Observations on pleural fluid pressure and volume relationships during therapeutic thoracentesis. The American review of respiratory disease. 1980;**121**(5):799–804

[20] Feller-Kopman D, Parker MJ, Schwartzstein RM. Assessment of pleural pressure in the evaluation of unexplained pleural effusions. Chest. 2004;**126**(6):2068–2073

[21] Lentz RJ, Lerner AD, Lahm T, et al. Pleural manometry during thoracentesis: A randomized trial. American journal of respiratory and critical care medicine. 2021;**203**:718–726

[22] West JB. Respiratory Physiology: The Essentials. 10th ed. Philadelphia: Lippincott Williams & Wilkins; 2016. p. 17–28

[23] Baumann MH, Strange C, Heffner JE, et al. Management of spontaneous pneumothorax: An American College of Chest Physicians Delphi consensus statement. Chest. 2001;**119**:590–602

[24] Sartori S, Tombesi P. Tension pneumothorax. European Journal of Internal Medicine. 2010;**21**(6):560–568

[25] Porcel JM. Pleural effusions from congestive heart failure. Current opinion in pulmonary medicine. 2013;**19**(4):357–364

[26] Hooper C, Lee YC, Maskell N. Investigation of a unilateral pleural effusion in adults: British Thoracic Society guideline. Thorax. 2010;**65** (Suppl 2):ii4–ii17

[27] Light RW. Clinical practice. New England Journal of Medicine. 2002;**346** (25):1971–1977

[28] Marik PE. Pleural Effusions and Atelectasis. In: Marik, PE. Evidence-Based Critical Care. Cham: Springer; 2015. p. 239–247. DOI: 10.1007/978-3-319-11020-2_26

[29] Bhatnagar M, Fisher A, Ramsaroop S, Carter A, Pippard B. Chylothorax: Pathophysiology, diagnosis, and management-a comprehensive review. Journal of Thoracic Disease. 2024;**16** (2):1645–1661. DOI: 10.21037/jtd-23-1636

[30] Antony VB, Loddenkemper R, Astoul P, et al. Management of malignant pleural effusions. European Respiratory Journal. 2001;**18**:402–419

[31] Mossman BT, Churg A. Mechanisms in the pathogenesis of asbestosis and silicosis. American Journal of Respiratory and Critical Care Medicine. 1998;**157**(5 Pt 1):1666–1680

Chapter 2

Breathing Between the Lines, Pleura Anatomy, Disorders and Clinical Insights

Basil Younis, Mohammad Alabdallat and Maricar Rulloda-Agoncillo

Abstract

The pleura, composed of visceral and parietal layers, is a vital serous membrane that envelops the lungs and lines the thoracic cavity. Its anatomical complexity and physiological function are central to standard respiratory mechanics and play a critical role in numerous clinical disorders. The visceral pleura is avascular and innervated by autonomic fibers, whereas the parietal pleura is richly supplied by systemic circulation and somatic nerves, making it highly sensitive to pain. Between these layers lies the pleural cavity, which contains a small volume of lubricating fluid that facilitates frictionless movement of the lungs during respiration. Pleural fluid homeostasis is maintained by mesothelial transport and lymphatic drainage, particularly through the parietal pleura. When this equilibrium is disrupted, pleural pathology results, frequently manifesting as empyema, pleural effusion, pneumothorax, hemothorax, or pleural cancer. Imaging, thoracentesis, and pleural fluid analysis are all parts of the diagnostic evaluation that inform clinical judgment and treatment. Understanding fluid dynamics, mesothelial biology, and minimally invasive management methods has improved significantly in recent years. Accurately diagnosing and treating pleural diseases requires a solid grasp of pleural anatomy and physiology. This chapter provides a comprehensive overview of the pleura's structural and functional features, thereby linking fundamental understanding with practical application.

Keywords: pleura, effusion, pneumothorax, mesothelioma, thoracentesis

1. Introduction

The pleura, a dynamic as well as metabolically active structure, plays an essential role in maintaining basic respiratory mechanics. Its anatomy and physiology are tightly regulated, and the disruption of these processes underlies a wide range of clinically significant pathologies [1–4].

The pleural space (PS) is a thin cavity located between the parietal and visceral pleura (VP), both of which are lined by a continuous layer of mesothelial cells

[2, 5–7]. While research on pleural fluid dynamics in healthy individuals is limited, available data suggest that pleural fluid is produced by systemic vessels in the pleural membranes at a rate of about 0.6 mL/hour and is absorbed at a similar rate by the parietal pleural lymphatic system [1, 8–10]. The PS usually contains a minimal volume, typically around 0.25 mL/kg of body weight, of low-protein fluid [5]. Despite its clinical importance often being underestimated, the pleura is far more than a simple anatomical partition. The PS serves as a dynamic interface that is integral to immunological defense, the regulation of fluid balance, and the mechanical efficiency of respiration.

This chapter begins with a foundational review of pleural anatomy and physiology, followed by an examination of major pleural pathologies. A central theme is the translation of fundamental pleural biology into clinical practice for both acute and chronic disease states, to reinforce evidence-based diagnostic and management strategies.

2. Pleural anatomy

2.1 The PS

The PS is a real (though extremely narrow) cavity, only 10–20 μm wide, wrapping entirely around the lungs up to the hilum [6, 8, 11]. The pulmonary architecture includes a dual-layered membrane system composed of the visceral and parietal pleura. The VP maintains intimate contact with the lung parenchyma and extends into the interlobar fissures. On the other hand, the parietal pleura forms a continuous lining along the thoracic wall, diaphragm, and mediastinum [2, 5, 6]. Each membrane covers a considerable surface area of approximately 1,000 cm^2 and receives vascular supply from the systemic circulation [2, 5, 12]. An essential anatomical difference distinguishing these layers is the lymphatic stomata, which are found exclusively within the parietal pleura. The stomata, measuring 2–6 μm in diameter, establish a direct conduit for fluid removal from the PS. This special anatomical arrangement is crucial in maintaining pleural fluid balance [13].

2.2 Parietal pleura: The fluid drainage hub

The parietal pleura plays a central role in fluid regulation due to the following:

- Its proximity to lymphatic stomata (which actively absorb fluid).
- Its consistent anatomy across species (unlike the variable VP).
- It has a rich systemic blood supply, which influences fluid production.

The mesothelial layer and the subpleural connective tissue layer, which contain intercostal arteries, nerves, and lymphatics, comprise the structurally 30–40 μm-thick parietal pleura [14]. Fluid exchange is facilitated by the microvessels in this region, which are only 10–12 μm from the PS.

Its most intriguing characteristic is the lymphatic stomata, which are tiny pores with a diameter of 2–6 μm that open directly into the PS [14, 15]. During inspiration, these stomata enlarge, improving drainage. They connect to underlying lymphatic "lakes" (lacunae) that eventually empty into larger lymph vessels, appearing as holes in the mesothelial layer under electron microscopy.

Studies in animals estimate 100–200 stomata per cm^2, with higher concentrations in dependent (lower) regions [14, 16, 17]. Remarkably, experiments show that red blood cells and carbon particles injected into the PS can enter these stomata and reach lymphatics within 15–30 minutes [14, 18].

2.3 VP: A structural support system

The VP varies in thickness (20–80 μm), being thickest near the lung base and thinnest at the apex [6, 19]. Unlike the parietal pleura, it lacks lymphatic stomata and instead contains the following:

- Bronchial artery capillaries (draining into pulmonary veins).
- Subpleural lymphatics (not connected to the PS).

This anatomy has two key implications as follows:

- Lower fluid production (due to lower pressure in pulmonary veins).
- Increased fluid leakage if pulmonary pressures rise (e.g., in heart failure).

Interestingly, small mammals (mice, rabbits) have much thinner VP (5–10 μm) without a bronchial blood supply, suggesting that, in larger species (like humans), the VP may help stabilize lung structure, prevent overexpansion, and distribute ventilation evenly.

2.4 Mesothelial cells: More than just a barrier

Mesothelial cells form the delicate lining of all the body's serous cavities (the pleura, pericardium, and peritoneum), where they play several essential roles [19, 20]. Fluid movement across the pleura is not an active, pumped process. Instead, mesothelial cells form a semi-permeable, "leaky" barrier that allows water and proteins to move passively, in a manner analogous to peritoneal dialysis.

On a microscopic level, pleural mesothelial cells are thin, squamous-like structures, measuring only 1–4 micrometers in thickness [21]. Yet, this delicate appearance is deceiving. These cells are metabolically active and structurally complex, containing a rich assortment of microtubules, microfilaments, vesicles, and other organelles [7, 19, 20]. A dense field of microvilli covers their luminal surface, greatly expanding their functional surface area [7, 19, 20].

These cells are far from being a passive lining; they are deeply involved in maintaining pleural homeostasis [7, 19]. They secrete key lubricating molecules, such as phospholipids and the large glycosaminoglycan hyaluronan, into the PS [22, 23]. This combination of substances ensures that the pleural surfaces can glide smoothly against each other during respiration, minimizing friction [22, 23]. Furthermore, they release a broad spectrum of signaling molecules – including chemokines, cytokines, and growth factors – that are critical for modulating inflammation and orchestrating tissue repair and remodeling after an injury [7].

To recap, the role of pleural mesothelial cells is complex. In addition to producing extracellular matrix to maintain tissue structure [24], they also act as phagocytes to clear cellular debris [25, 85]. Their regulatory functions are equally important, as they can orchestrate inflammatory responses by releasing cytokines and recruiting immune cells [26–29]. They are critical in maintaining the balance between coagulation and fibrinolysis, a function that prevents the formation of abnormal clots within the PS [30, 31].

3. Pleural physiologies

3.1 Pleural excursion

When the respiratory system reaches functional residual capacity (FRC), pleural pressure stabilizes at approximately -6 cm H_2O [5, 8, 12]. This negative intrapleural pressure reflects a balance between the lungs' inherent tendency to collapse inward and the chest wall's natural inclination to expand outward [5, 8, 9, 12]. Additionally, gravity creates a vertical pressure gradient of roughly 0.2 cm H_2O per centimeter of lung height [12, 32]. During the inspiratory phase, the diaphragm and external intercostal muscles contract, which expands the thoracic cavity and causes pleural pressure to drop further [5, 9, 12]. This reduction in pressure creates a negative gradient across the alveolar membrane, drawing air into the respiratory system. Expiration, however, is a fundamentally different process that primarily occurs through passive mechanisms. As the diaphragm and inspiratory muscles relax, the elastic properties of the lung tissue, working together with the chest wall's outward tension, produce a modest elevation in pleural pressure that facilitates air expulsion. However, it remains subatmospheric (about –3 to –5 cm H_2O at FRC) [5, 8, 12]. This persistently negative pleural pressure is crucial for maintaining lung inflation [5, 8, 12]. When it is lost – as in pneumothorax or with a large pleural effusion – the unopposed elastic recoil of the lung causes collapse [1, 33, 34].

3.2 Pleural fluid dynamics

The balance of hydrostatic and oncotic pressures across the pleural membranes governs the dynamics of pleural fluid. Fluid is primarily produced by filtration from the systemic capillaries of the parietal pleura, driven by higher hydrostatic pressure relative to the VP. At the same time, resorption occurs mainly via lymphatic stomata (cylindrical-like openings with a diameter of 0.5 to 20.0 mm, which are formed by discontinuities in the parietal mesothelium and submesothelial interstitial space) [35, 36], particularly in the diaphragmatic and mediastinal regions [1, 9]. The pleural lymphatic system is the most critical mechanism for quantitatively removing pleural fluid and can increase its drainage capacity up to 20-fold in response to increased fluid formation [1, 10]. The negative intrapleural pressure (typically -3 to -5 cm H_2O at FRC) is essential for lung expansion. It is maintained by the opposing elastic recoil forces of the lung and chest wall [1, 10].

3.2.1 Formation

Studies (mostly in sheep, which have similar pleural anatomy to humans) suggest the following:

- Normal pleural fluid volume: ~0.1–0.2 mL/kg (in humans, ~8.4 mL per hemithorax) [37].
- Composition: low protein (~1 g/dL), few white blood cells (mostly macrophages).
- Production rate: 0.6 mL/hour (from systemic vessels, not pulmonary circulation) [13].

3.2.2 Why systemic vessels?

- Higher pressure → more filtration.
- Closer proximity to the PS.
- Lower protein content in pleural fluid matches systemic capillary filtrate (unlike pulmonary filtrate, which is protein-rich).

The parietal pleura likely contributes more fluid than the VP because of the following:

- Its microvessels are closer to the PS.
- Its drainage pressure is higher (visceral fluid drains into low-pressure pulmonary veins).

3.2.3 Absorption (fluid clearance)

Under normal conditions, fluid is absorbed at the same rate it is produced (0.6 mL/hour). However, if excess fluid accumulates, drainage can increase 10-fold (up to 0.28 mL/kg per hour) [13, 38].

3.2.4 Key evidence for lymphatic drainage

- Protein concentration stays constant during absorption (suggesting bulk flow, not diffusion).
- Red blood cells exit intact (only possible through stomata).
- No active transport by mesothelial cells (pleural pressure is lower than tissue pressure, favoring inward flow).

3.2.5 Lymphatic flow (the final drainage pathway)

Lymphatic drainage is boosted by the following:

- Intrinsic contractions (regulated by hormones/nerves) [39].
- Respiratory movements (expanding stomata during inspiration) [39].
- Fluid circulation within the PS [32, 40].

4. Pleural pathology

Pleural diseases are categorized into congenital and acquired disorders (see **Table 1**).

4.1 Congenital pleural diseases

Congenital pleural diseases are rare congenital disabilities of development. They often present with lymphatic malformations predisposing to chyle effusion, but structural abnormalities and genetic syndromes can also adversely affect pleural architecture. Early antenatal diagnosis and immediate postnatal care are essential for lowering the risks of neonatal respiratory morbidity [33, 41].

4.1.1 Congenital chylothorax

Definition: Perinatal accumulation of chyle in the PS secondary to nondevelopment, obstruction, or spontaneous rupture of the thoracic duct or its principal lymphatic tributaries [42–45]. It is the primary etiology of neonatal pleural effusion [42, 44, 46].

Epidemiology: The estimated incidence is approximately 1 in 10,000–24,000 live births; a male predominance is reported in some series [42]. It may be isolated or associated with lymphatic dysplasia (e.g., generalized lymphatic anomaly) or chromosomal disorders [47].

Pathophysiology: Chyle arises from intestinal lymph and contains triglyceride-rich chylomicrons and lymphocytes [43]. Leakage into the PS leads to respiratory compromise and nutritional/immunological depletion.

Clinical features: Fetal hydrops, mediastinal shift on antenatal ultrasound, and postnatal respiratory distress [44]. Effusions are often bilateral; right-sided predominance is frequent due to thoracic duct anatomy.

Category		Examples	Key features/notes
Congenital		Congenital chylothorax, fetal hydrothorax, lymphangiomatosis, congenital pleural cyst	Present at birth or early infancy; often associated with lymphatic abnormalities
Acquired	Traumatic	Blunt chest trauma, penetrating injury, iatrogenic, traumatic chylothorax	History of injury or procedure may cause pneumothorax, hemothorax, or chylothorax
	Nontraumatic	Spontaneous pneumothorax, pleural effusion, pleural infection, pleural tumors, others	No trauma history; related to underlying pulmonary, cardiac, renal, malignant, or systemic disease

Table 1.
Based on the author's synthesis of current knowledge.

Investigations: Ultrasound confirms effusion. Performing a diagnostic thoracentesis will demonstrate milky fluid with triglycerides typically ≥1.24 mmol/L (≥110 mg/dL) after enteral feeding and lymphocyte predominance [48]. Consider biochemical testing for triglycerides and chylomicrons.

Management: Conservative therapy (drainage if required, medium-chain triglyceride [MCT] formula or fat-free feeds, total parenteral nutrition when needed) is the first line of treatment [45]. Pharmacological reduction of lymph flow with octreotide is widely used [49]. Refractory cases may require thoracic duct ligation or pleurodesis [50]. Multidisciplinary care, including neonatology, pediatric surgery, and nutrition, is essential.

Clinical pearl: Withholding long-chain triglycerides and using MCT-based feeds can substantially reduce chyle production and accelerate the resolution of chyle leakage.

4.1.2 Congenital (fetal/neonatal) pleural effusion (hydrothorax)

Definition: Pleural fluid accumulation is recognized antenatally or within the first 28 days of life [51]. Primary fetal hydrothorax typically reflects lymphatic leakage. On the other hand, secondary fetal hydrothorax causes include congenital infections and cardiac anomalies.

Assessment and management: To assess and monitor the size and hydrops, serial antenatal ultrasounds should be performed [52]. In severe cases, intrauterine thoracentesis or thoracoamniotic shunting must be considered [53]. Postnatally, management includes stabilizing the airway, draining large effusions, and evaluating for chylothorax and secondary causes [54].

4.1.3 Other rare congenital pleural disorders

Pleural lymphangiomatosis and benign pleural cysts are some rare congenital pleural disorders [55], which are managed in an individualized manner and are often supportive.

4.2 Acquired pleural diseases

4.2.1 Traumatic

Traumatic pleural diseases result from either direct or indirect injury to the pleura, which leads to the accumulation of air, blood, chyle, or other fluids in the PS [56]. Traumatic injuries may be penetrating, blunt, or iatrogenic [56–61], with clinical consequences depending on the mechanism, extent of injury, and associated intrathoracic or extrathoracic damage.

4.2.1.1 Blunt and penetrating trauma

Blunt trauma, such as from motor vehicle collisions or falls, is the common cause of pneumothorax and hemothorax [57]. Penetrating trauma, including stab wounds and gunshot injuries, carries a high risk of direct pleural breach and associated vascular injury [58]. Blunt trauma, usually caused by rib fractures lacerating the pleura, contributes to the majority of cases, while penetrating trauma, blast injuries, or barotrauma make up the remainder.

4.2.1.1.1 Pneumothorax

The underlying pathophysiology is the loss of negative intrapleural pressure, leading to partial or complete lung collapse. Depending on the mechanism, patients may present with a simple pneumothorax, a tension variant with mediastinal shift and obstructive shock, or an open pneumothorax with direct communication to the atmosphere.

Clinically, patients develop sudden pleuritic chest pain, dyspnea, tachypnea, and reduced breath sounds on the affected side [62], as well as signs such as hyperresonance and subcutaneous emphysema. Tension pneumothorax is a life-threatening emergency marked by severe respiratory distress, hypotension, distended neck veins, and tracheal deviation [34, 63, 64].

Diagnosis is mainly radiological. An upright chest X-ray reveals a visible pleural line with absent peripheral markings, while supine trauma films may show the deep sulcus sign [3, 34, 64].

Computed tomography (CT) offers the most sensitive detection, especially for occult cases, and point-of-care ultrasound is increasingly valuable, as demonstrated by the absence of lung sliding on M-mode. Performing Extended Focused Assessment with Sonography for Trauma (eFAST) is helpful in unstable patients [65].

Management of traumatic pneumothorax follows the principles of Advanced Trauma Life Support (ATLS), addressing life-threatening conditions during the primary survey. The goals are prompt lung re-expansion, prevention of recurrence, and treatment of associated injuries.

Tension pneumothorax is an emergency that requires immediate needle decompression, traditionally performed at the second intercostal space, mid-clavicular line; however, the fourth or fifth intercostal space at the anterior axillary line is now preferred for reliability [34, 63, 64]. Insertion of a chest tube thoracostomy is usually performed afterward [34, 63, 64].

For simple traumatic pneumothorax, such as small and stable cases, conservative management is preferred, involving oxygen therapy, observation, and repeat imaging [34, 61, 65]. With larger or symptomatic pneumothoraces, a tube thoracostomy should be inserted at the fifth intercostal space in the mid-axillary line [34, 61, 65].

In open pneumothorax, also known as "sucking chest wounds," initial stabilization is achieved with a three-sided occlusive dressing to prevent further air entry while allowing egress [34, 63]. This is followed by chest tube insertion at a separate site and definitive surgical repair of the defect [34, 63].

4.2.1.1.2 Hemithorax

Traumatic hemothorax complicates nearly one-third of significant blunt and penetrating chest injuries, most often resulting from motor vehicle collisions, falls, or violence-related stab and gunshot wounds. Mortality is usually determined by associated injuries rather than the hemothorax itself.

The pathogenesis reflects injury to the thoracic structures, such as blunt trauma, which causes rib fractures and laceration of intercostal vessels or lung parenchyma, while penetrating mechanisms directly disrupt intercostal, internal mammary, or pulmonary vessels. Accumulated blood within the PS compresses the lung, reduces ventilation, and may precipitate hypovolemic shock. Failure to evacuate it promptly risks the development of fibrothorax.

Clinically, patients present with dyspnea, chest pain, and hypovolemic features such as tachycardia, dizziness, or hypotension. Examination will reveal absent breath sounds and dullness to percussion over the affected hemithorax. Large bleeds can sometimes mimic the physiology of a tamponade, which is characterized by distension of the neck veins. Hemothoraces are classified by volume: minimal (<350 mL, often resolving on its own), moderate (350–1,500 mL, usually requiring tube drainage), and massive (>1,500 mL initially or >200 mL/h ongoing), which will mandate urgent surgical exploration.

In practice, tube thoracostomy serves as both a diagnostic and therapeutic procedure, with the initial drainage volume guiding classification and management.

The management of traumatic hemothorax centers on restoring adequate ventilation, controlling hemorrhage, and preventing late complications such as fibrothorax or empyema. Initial care is based on the principles of ATLS, ensuring airway patency, oxygen delivery, intravenous access, fluid resuscitation, and early blood typing and cross-matching.

Tube thoracostomy is the cornerstone of treatment. A large-bore (28–32 Fr) chest tube is inserted in the fifth intercostal space at the mid-axillary line and connected to an underwater seal system to evacuate blood, re-expand the lung, and monitor ongoing losses [56, 61].

A massive hemothorax is defined as immediate drainage exceeding 1,500 mL of blood or an output of more than 200 mL per hour for four consecutive hours. These thresholds indicate active bleeding and mandate urgent thoracotomy to control hemorrhage and repair injured vessels [56, 61]. In selected stable patients with retained clot or persistent collections, video-assisted thoracoscopic surgery (VATS) provides a minimally invasive option for evacuation, decortication, and prevention of sequelae [61].

Clinical pearl: In trauma, suspect occult pneumothorax in patients with subcutaneous emphysema, even if the chest radiograph appears normal [61, 65].

4.2.1.2 Iatrogenic pleural injury

Iatrogenic injury is increasingly recognized due to the rising number of thoracic and non-thoracic procedures [59]. Common causes include central venous catheterization, transthoracic needle biopsy, thoracentesis, and mechanical ventilation (barotrauma).

Incidence: Pneumothorax occurs in up to 20% of transthoracic needle biopsies [60]. The use of real-time ultrasound guidance has reduced complication rates in thoracentesis [66].

Management principles mirror those for trauma-related pneumothorax and hemothorax, with added emphasis on prevention via image guidance and adherence to procedural safety protocols.

Clinical pearl: Always perform post-procedural imaging after high-risk interventions to detect delayed pneumothorax.

4.2.1.3 Traumatic chylothorax

Traumatic causes for chylothorax account for up to 25% overall. This may be due to the traumatic disruption of the thoracic duct from either a penetrating trauma or a surgical injury (notably esophagectomy) [67]. Its diagnosis relies on pleural fluid analysis, which will yield triglycerides ≥1.24 mmol/L (≥110 mg/dL) and the presence of chylomicrons [68].

Management: Drainage, dietary modification (MCT diet or nil per os with parenteral nutrition), and octreotide are some of the initial conservative interventions [69]. Surgical ligation of the thoracic duct or pleuroperitoneal shunting should be considered for persistent high-output leaks [42, 43, 50, 69].

Clinical pearl: In post-esophagectomy patients with persistent chest drain output of milky fluid, always consider chylothorax as a potential diagnosis.

4.2.1.4 Traumatic empyema

Uncommon but serious complication of chest trauma, more frequent after penetrating injuries or retained hemothorax.

Incidence: ~2–4% of all chest trauma admissions, which may be higher if chest tubes are delayed or poorly positioned.

4.2.1.4.1 Primary causes

Direct inoculation: Penetrating trauma introduces bacteria directly into the PS.

Secondary infection: May be due to infected and retained hemothorax or pneumothorax fluid [61].

Iatrogenic: Occurs as an infection post-tube thoracostomy, thoracoscopy, or other pleural procedures.

4.2.1.4.2 Pathophysiology

Pleural space infection progresses through three stages [70]:

- Exudative phase: Inflammatory cells are found in the sterile fluid.
- Fibro-purulent phase: Bacterial invasion, pus formation, fibrin deposition, septation.
- Organizing phase: Fibroblast ingrowth, trapped lung, chronic empyema.

4.2.1.4.3 Symptoms

Symptoms are characterized by fever, chills, night sweats, pleuritic chest pain, dyspnea, and productive cough if there is parenchymal involvement.

4.2.1.4.4 Signs

Signs may show decreased breath sounds, dullness to percussion, local tenderness over the trauma site, and occasionally purulent drainage from the tube site.

4.2.1.4.5 Diagnostic approach

Laboratory: Complete blood count (CBC) will show leukocytosis. Elevated C-reactive protein (CRP) and erythrocyte sedimentation rate (ESR) are also common.

Pleural fluid analysis (diagnostic thoracentesis): The gross appearance will be turbid or purulent. A pH <7.2, glucose <60 mg/dL, lactate dehydrogenase (LDH) > 1000 IU/L strongly suggest infection. Gram stain or culture will be positive [71].

Imaging: Chest X-ray will show homogeneous opacity, often loculated.

Ultrasound: This detects septations and guides drainage.

CT chest scan: This defines the extent and detects associated lung abscesses.

4.2.1.4.6 Management

Antibiotics: Start empirically (cover Gram-positive cocci, Gram-negative bacilli, anaerobes) and adjust according to culture results.

Drainage: Tube thoracostomy for free-flowing pus. An image-guided pigtail catheter is possible for small loculations.

Intrapleural fibrinolysis: Tissue plasminogen activator (tPA) + deoxyribonuclease (DNase) to break septations in the fibro-purulent stage.

Surgical intervention: VATS for multiloculated or organizing empyema. For trapped lungs, an open thoracotomy/decortication should be performed.

4.2.2 Nontraumatic

Without any direct external or iatrogenic injury to the pleura, nontraumatic pleural diseases can occur and usually result from either primary pleural pathology or secondary involvement in systemic or intrathoracic disease [1]. This kind of injury may result from a spontaneous pneumothorax to malignant pleural involvement, with varying etiologies, presentations, and management approaches.

4.2.2.1 Spontaneous pneumothorax

Epidemiology: Incidence (per 100,000/year) – primary spontaneous pneumothorax (PSP) ≈ 7–18 in men, 2–6 in women; secondary spontaneous pneumothorax (SSP) ≈ 3–6 in men, 1–2 in women.

Spontaneous pneumothorax occurs without antecedent trauma and is categorized as primary (no underlying lung disease) or secondary (associated with lung pathology) [34]. Primary spontaneous pneumothorax (PSP) typically affects tall, thin young men and is linked to subpleural bleb rupture [72]. Secondary spontaneous pneumothorax (SSP) is most commonly caused by chronic obstructive pulmonary disease (COPD), interstitial lung disease, and infections such as Pneumocystis jirovecii [73].

The classification is presented in **Table 2**.

BTS 2023 guidance recommends initial conservative management for stable PSP with minimal symptoms, as spontaneous resolution is standard [64]. Needle aspiration or intercostal drainage is indicated for larger or symptomatic PSP and for most SSP cases.

Clinical pearl: Always exclude secondary causes in patients over 50 presenting with an apparent "primary" spontaneous pneumothorax.

4.2.2.2 Pleural effusion

Pleural effusion is the abnormal accumulation of fluid in the PS, classified as transudate or exudate according to Light's criteria [74] (see **Table 3**). Common

Type	Definition/features	Pathogenesis and risk factors
Primary spontaneous pneumothorax (PSP)	Occurs without clinically apparent lung disease; most commonly due to the rupture of apical subpleural blebs or bullae. Typically seen in young, tall, thin males	• Microscopic airway inflammation and subpleural blebs/bullae rupture with pressure swings • Smoking: a major, dose-dependent risk factor (increases risk × 22 in men, × 9 in women) • Genetic predispositions: Birt–Hogg–Dubé syndrome (FLCN mutation), Marfan syndrome, alpha-1 antitrypsin deficiency
Secondary spontaneous pneumothorax (SSP)	Occurs in patients with underlying lung disease, for example: • COPD/emphysema (most common) • Cystic lung diseases: LAM, Birt–Hogg–Dubé • Interstitial lung disease (fibrosis, sarcoidosis) • Infections: TB, PCP, necrotizing pneumonia, COVID-related cysts • Cystic fibrosis	• Air leaks through diseased, fragile lung parenchyma • Greater physiological impact due to already reduced respiratory reserve • Risk factors: older age, advanced underlying disease, ventilatory support
Catamenial pneumothorax	Recurrent PSP occurring within 72 hours of menstruation; strong right-sided predominance, due to thoracic endometriosis	• Diaphragmatic fenestrations or pleural implants allow air or endometrial tissue translocation into the pleural space • The risk of recurrence is high unless hormonal and surgical therapy is considered

Table 2.
Based on the author's synthesis of current knowledge.

Criterion	Exudate	Transudate
Pleural fluid protein/serum protein	> 0.5	≤0.5
Pleural fluid LDH/serum LDH	>0.6	≤0.6
Pleural fluid LDH (absolute value)	>2/3 upper limit of normal for serum LDH	≤2/3 ULN

Table 3.
Light's criteria for pleural effusion [70].

causes of transudates include heart failure, cirrhosis, and nephrotic syndrome, while exudates are usually caused by pneumonia, malignancy, or tuberculosis (TB) [75] (see **Table 4**).

The cornerstone of evaluating a pleural effusion is performing a diagnostic thoracentesis with pleural fluid analysis. BTS 2023 guidelines emphasize the role of thoracic ultrasound before aspiration to reduce complications [76]. Management targets the underlying cause and may involve therapeutic drainage.

Clinical pearl: A "borderline" Light's criteria result in a patient on diuretics may still represent a transudate. Consider serum–pleural albumin gradient.

Type		Common Causes	Notes
Transudate		Heart failure, cirrhosis, nephrotic syndrome, hypoalbuminemia	Low protein; treat underlying cause
Exudate	Infective	Parapneumonic effusion, tuberculosis, empyema	High protein; may require drainage
	Malignant	Lung cancer, breast cancer, lymphoma, mesothelioma	Often recurrent; consider pleurodesis or IPC
	Other	Pulmonary embolism, autoimmune (RA, SLE), pancreatitis, post-CABG	Varied presentation; targeted therapy

Table 4.
Based on the author's synthesis of current knowledge.

4.2.2.3 Pleural infection (empyema)

Empyema is a purulent pleural effusion that typically follows pneumonia, thoracic surgery, or esophageal rupture [64]. The pathogenesis involves progression from an exudative to a fibrinopurulent and then an organizing stage [70].

The 2023 BTS guidelines advocate for the early use of intrapleural fibrinolytic therapy (tPA and DNase) in patients with loculated empyema who are unresponsive to initial drainage [77]. Surgical referral is warranted if medical management fails.

Clinical pearl: Intrapleural tPA + DNase has been shown to improve drainage and reduce surgical referral rates [77].

4.2.2.4 Pleural tumors

4.2.2.4.1 Benign pleural tumors

- Solitary fibrous tumor
- Pleural lipoma
- Pleural thickening and fibrosis: Pleural thickening may result from chronic inflammation, infection, or asbestos exposure.
- Diffuse pleural thickening can restrict lung expansion and cause dyspnea.
- Pleural fibrosis is often irreversible and may be associated with calcification [78].
- Pleural calcifications are typically benign and associated with prior infections or asbestos exposure.
- Pleural plaques are the hallmark of asbestos exposure and are usually asymptomatic.
- A prior empyema or hemothorax can result in extensive calcification [79].

4.2.2.4.2 Malignant pleural disease

Malignant pleural diseases are considered a significant clinical challenge due to their insidious onset, diagnostic complexity, and poor prognosis. These conditions may arise from primary pleural tumors or secondary involvement from metastatic malignancies. Early recognition and accurate differentiation from benign pleural processes are needed for timely intervention and improved outcomes. Malignant pleural diseases are often due to metastatic spread, usually from lung and breast carcinoma, and mesothelioma [80].

4.2.2.4.2.1 Malignant pleural effusion

Malignant pleural effusion (MPE) is a common manifestation of advanced malignancy, occurring in approximately 15% of all cancer patients [81].

- Clinical features include progressive dyspnea, chest discomfort, and cough.
- Diagnosis is made through cytological analysis of pleural fluid or pleural biopsy.
- Management includes therapeutic thoracentesis, indwelling pleural catheters (IPCs), and pleurodesis.

4.2.2.4.2.2 Primary pleural tumors

The most notable primary pleural malignancy is malignant mesothelioma, which is strongly associated with asbestos exposure.

- Histological subtypes include epithelioid, sarcomatoid, and biphasic.
- Latency period may exceed 30 years post-exposure.
- Nonspecific symptoms may include chest pain, weight loss, and pleural effusion.
- Prognosis is poor, with a median survival of 9 to 18 months [82].

4.2.2.4.2.3 Secondary pleural involvement

Metastatic spread to the pleura is usually more common than primary pleural tumors with the frequent sources being lung and breast cancers. Mechanisms include direct extension, hematogenous spread, or lymphatic dissemination.

Image-guided biopsy or thoracoscopy is often required for diagnosis.

BTS 2023 guidelines recommend IPC or talc pleurodesis for recurrent malignant effusions, with the patient's preference being considered [83]. Parallel systemic therapy with local control measures should be optimized together.

Clinical pearl: IPCs enable the outpatient management of recurrent malignant effusions, thereby improving quality of life.

4.2.2.5 Other nontraumatic pleural disorders

Autoimmune pleuritis (e.g., lupus, rheumatoid arthritis [RA]), drug-induced pleural disease (e.g., nitrofurantoin, amiodarone), and postcardiac injury syndrome are other causes of nontraumatic pleural disorders [84], wherein management will depend on its etiology and often involves immunosuppression.

5. Conclusion

The pleura, a dynamic serous membrane, has anatomical and physiological integrity that is fundamental to respiratory mechanics. This comprehensive review assimilates foundational science with clinical pathology to highlight its significance in a broad spectrum of diseases [1, 2, 41].

A thorough understanding of pleural pathophysiology is founded on its unique anatomical and physiological features. The structural contrast between the visceral and parietal pleura, specifically the restriction of lymphatic stomata to the parietal surface, is the primary determinant of pleural fluid dynamics [13, 14]. The negative intrapleural pressure, resulting from the opposing elastic recoil of the lung and chest wall, is fundamental for maintaining lung inflation [5, 8, 12]. At the cellular level, the mesothelial cell functions not as a passive barrier but as a metabolically active unit that secretes lubricating molecules and modulates local inflammatory and fibrinolytic processes [19, 22, 23, 30, 31].

Pleural diseases encompass a broad spectrum, ranging from congenital malformations to acquired conditions – whether traumatic, iatrogenic, infectious, inflammatory, or neoplastic. Disruptions to this homeostasis result in a wide range of clinical pathologies. Congenital anomalies, such as chylothorax, highlight the importance of lymphatic integrity [42, 46]. Acquired conditions, including traumatic hemopneumothorax, necessitate emergent interventions to restore negative intrapleural pressure and achieve hemodynamic stability [61, 63, 64]. In the context of pleural infection, the progression from a simple parapneumonic effusion to a complex empyema demonstrates the pleura's active immunological role [70]. The efficacy of intrapleural fibrinolytic therapy with tPA and DNase exemplifies a targeted, pathophysiology-based treatment strategy that can prevent the need for surgical intervention [77]. For MPE, management has advanced, prioritizing palliative strategies, such as IPC, in alignment with established clinical practice guidelines [78, 83].

Their presentations usually range from asymptomatic effusions to life-threatening pneumothoraxes, as well as malignant pleural syndromes. Understanding the underlying pleural dynamics, such as the balance between hydrostatic, oncotic, and lymphatic forces, is needed, as it explains the genesis of effusions. At the same time, the disruption of negative intrapleural pressure underpins the pathophysiology of pneumothorax.

Imaging advances, such as [3, 66], thoracoscopy, molecular microbiology [71], and pleural manometry, have refined diagnostic accuracy. Modern imaging modalities, molecular diagnostics, and minimally invasive techniques have collectively enhanced diagnostic accuracy and therapeutic efficacy [3, 66, 71]. Evolving guidelines in trauma [61], infection [64], and oncology [79, 83] have improved patient outcomes. The combination of these technologies with an evidence-based approach, as mirrored in contemporary clinical guidelines for trauma, infection, and oncology, has led to improved patient outcomes [61, 64, 83].

Management strategies now emphasize minimally invasive interventions, such as VATS [61], IPCs [83], and image-guided procedures [66], while adhering to core principles of stabilization and restoration of respiratory function.

Ultimately, pleural diseases emphasize the pleura as both a mirror and mediator of systemic health [1, 41]. A comprehensive understanding of anatomy and physiology, as well as the dynamics of the pleura, provides the foundation for accurate diagnosis, rational management, and prevention of long-term sequelae [1, 2, 41]. Integrating knowledge with modern advances guarantees improved care for patients with pleural pathology. Continued research into the molecular and cellular mechanisms of pleural disease holds the promise of further innovation and will be essential for developing novel diagnostic and therapeutic strategies [1, 64, 83].

Acronyms and abbreviations

ACR	American College of Radiology
ATLS	Advanced Trauma Life Support
BTS	British Thoracic Society
CABG	Coronary artery bypass graft
CBC	Complete blood count
COPD	Chronic obstructive pulmonary disease
COVID	Coronavirus disease
CRP	C-reactive protein
CT	Computed tomography
DNase	Deoxyribonuclease
eFAST	Extended Focused Assessment with Sonography for Trauma
ESR	Erythrocyte sedimentation rate
FLCN	Folliculin
FRC	Functional residual capacity
IPC	Indwelling pleural catheter
LAM	Lymphangioleiomyomatosis
LDH	Lactate dehydrogenase
MCT	Medium-chain triglyceride
MPE	Malignant pleural effusion
NCCN	National Comprehensive Cancer Network
PCP	Pneumocystis pneumonia
PS	Pleural space
PSP	Primary spontaneous pneumothorax
RA	Rheumatoid arthritis
SLE	Systemic lupus erythematosus
SSP	Secondary spontaneous pneumothorax
TB	Tuberculosis
tPA	Tissue plasminogen activator
ULN	Upper limit of normal
VATS	Video-assisted thoracoscopic surgery
VP	Visceral pleura

DOI: http://dx.doi.org/10.5772/intechopen.1014968

Acknowledgments

The author gratefully acknowledges the support of Hamad Medical Corporation, Doha, Qatar, for providing the institutional framework and clinical resources necessary for the completion of this chapter. Special thanks are extended to the colleagues and staff of the Department of Thoracic and Trauma Surgery for their invaluable assistance and collaboration throughout this chapter.

The author also wishes to thank Dr. Hasan Al-Thani (Head of Trauma and Vascular Surgery) for guidance in writing this chapter, Dr. Talat Chughtai (Senior Consultant in Thoracic Surgery) for assistance with data collection, whose contributions significantly enriched the quality of this research, and Dr. Sandro Rizoli (Chief of Trauma Section) for his sharp insight and continuous encouragement to reach a high level of performance.

We would like to acknowledge the use of Grammarly in helping refine the language and clarity of this research. It was a useful tool for catching any typographical errors, improving sentence flow, as well as enhancing overall readability. However, all final edits and decisions were made by the authors to ensure the integrity of the content remained intact.

Conflict of Interest

I make the following declaration in relation to this chapter:

- There is no conflict of interest.
- The content is balanced and free of bias, whether commercial or noncommercial.
- This complies with the general health standards.
- There is no plagiarism or copyright infringement.

Author details

Basil Younis*, Mohammad Alabdallat and Maricar Rulloda-Agoncillo
Hamad Medical Corporation, Doha, Qatar

*Address all correspondence to: byounis@hamad.qa

References

[1] Feller-Kopman D, Light R. Pleural disease. New England Journal of Medicine. 2018;**378**:740–751. DOI: 10.1056/NEJMra1403503

[2] DeBiasi EM, Feller-Kopman D. Leading Journal, Anatomy and Applied Physiology of the Pleural Space. Clinics in Chest Medicine. 2021, **42** (4), 567–576. DOI: 10.1016/j.ccm.2021.08.005

[3] Diagnosis YA, Taiji R, Nishimoto Y, et al. Pictorial review of pleural disease: Multimodality imaging and differential. Radiographics: A Review Publication of the Radiological Society of North America, Inc. 2024;**44**(4):e230079. DOI: 10.1148/rg.230079

[4] Jones JS. The pleura in health and disease. Lung. 2001;**179**(6):397–413. DOI: 10.1007/s004080000075

[5] Broaddus VC. Chapter 14. Pleural Physiology and Pathophysiology. In: Murray and Nadel's Textbook of Respiratory Medicine Philadelphia. 7th ed. Elsevier; 2021. p. 180–195

[6] Wang NS. Anatomy of the pleura. In: Antony VB, editor. Diseases of the Pleura. Philadelphia: WB Saunders; 1998. p. 229

[7] Mutsaers SE. Mesothelial cells: Their structure, function, and role in serosal repair. Respirology. 2002;7(3):171–191

[8] Lai-Fook SJ. Pleural mechanics and fluid exchange. Physiological Reviews. 2004;**84**(2):385

[9] Physiology of the Pleural Space, C YA, Lazaridis G, et al. Charalampidis. Journal of Thoracic Disease. 2015;7 (Suppl 1)S33–7. DOI: 10.3978/j.issn.2072-1439.2014.12.48

[10] Negrini D, Moriondo A. Pleural Function and Lymphatics. Acta Physiologica (Oxford, England). 2013;**207**(2):244–259. DOI: 10.1111/apha.12016

[11] Albertine KH, Wiener-Kronish JP, Bastacky J. No evidence for mesothelial cell contact across the costal pleural space of sheep. Journal of Applied Physiology. 1991;**70**(1):123

[12] Agostoni E. Mechanics of the pleural space. Physiological Reviews. 1972;**52**(1):57–128

[13] Broaddus VC, Wiener-Kronish JP, Berthiaume Y, Staub NC. Removal of Pleural Liquid and Protein by Lymphatics in Awake Sheep. Journal of Applied Physiology. 1988;**64**(1):384–390. DOI: 10.1152/jappl.1988.64.1.384

[14] Albertine KH, Wiener-Kronish JP. The structure of the parietal pleura and its relationship to pleural liquid dynamics in sheep. The Anatomical Record. 1984;**208**(3):401

[15] Li J. Ultrastructural study on the pleural stomata in human. Funct Dev Morphol. 1993, **3** (4), 2

[16] Shinohara H. Distribution of lymphatic stomata on the pleural surface of the thoracic cavity and the surface topography of the pleural mesothelium in the golden hamster. The Anatomical Record. 1997;**249**(1):16

[17] Wang NS. The preformed stomata connecting the pleural cavity and the lymphatics in the parietal pleura. The

American Review of Respiratory Disease. 1975;**111**(1):12

[18] Miura T, Shimada T, Tanaka K, Chujo M, Uchida Y. Lymphatic drainage of carbon particles injected into the pleural cavity of the monkey, as studied by video-assisted thoracoscopy and electron microscopy. The Journal of Thoracic and Cardiovascular Surgery. 2000;**120**(3):437

[19] Mutsaers SE, Wilkosz S. Structure and function of mesothelial cells. Cancer Treatment and Research. 2007;**134**:120. Pathophysiology of the pleura. Jantz, MA, Antony, V.B. Respiration. 2008;75(2):121.

[20] Junqueira LC, Carneiro J. Junqueira's Basic Histology: Text & Atlas New York, USA. 15th ed. McGraw-Hill; 2018

[21] Wang NS. The regional difference of pleural mesothelial cells in rabbits. The American Review of Respiratory Disease. 1974;**110**(5):623–633

[22] Wang PM, Lai-Fook SJ. Pleural tissue hyaluronan produced by postmortem ventilation in rabbits. Lung. 2000;**178**(1):1–12

[23] Mills PC, Chen Y, Hills YC, et al. Comparison of surfactant lipids between pleural and pulmonary lining fluids. Pulmonary Pharmacology & Therapeutics. 2006;**19**:292–296

[24] Rennard SI, Jaurand MC, Bignon J, Kawanami O, Ferrans VJ, Davidson J, Crystal RG. Role of pleural mesothelial cells in the production of the submesothelial connective tissue matrix of the lung. American Review of Respiratory Disease. 1984;**130**(2):267

[25] Jaurand MC, Kaplan H, Thiollet J, Pinchon MC, Bernaudin JF. Phagocytosis of chrysotile fibers by pleural mesothelial cells in culture. The American Journal of Pathology. 1979;**94**(3):529

[26] Boylan AM, Rüegg C, Kim KJ, Hébert CA, Hoeffel JM, Pytela R, Sheppard D, Goldstein IM, Broaddus VC. Evidence of a role for mesothelial cell-derived interleukin 8 in the pathogenesis of asbestos-induced pleurisy in rabbits. Journal of Clinical Investigation. 1992;**89**(4):1257

[27] Jonjić N, Peri G, Bernasconi S, Sciacca FL, Colotta F, Pelicci P, Lanfrancone L, Mantovani A. Expression of adhesion molecules and chemotactic cytokines in cultured human mesothelial cells. The Journal of Experimental Medicine. 1992;**176**(4):1165

[28] Nasreen N, Mohammed KA, Hardwick J, Van Horn RD, Sanders KL, Doerschuk CM, Hott JW, Antony VB. Polar production of interleukin-8 by mesothelial cells promotes the transmesothelial migration of neutrophils: Role of intercellular adhesion molecule-1. The Journal of Infectious Diseases. 2001;**183**(11):1638

[29] Kuwahara M, Kuwahara M, Bijwaard KE, Gersten DM, Diglio CA, Kagan E. Mesothelial cells produce a chemoattractant for lung fibroblasts: Role of fibronectin. American Journal of Respiratory Cell and Molecular Biology. 1991;**5**(3):256

[30] Idell S, Zwieb C, Kumar A, Koenig KB, Johnson AR. Pathways of fibrin turnover of human pleural mesothelial cells in vitro. American Journal of Respiratory Cell and Molecular Biology. 1992;**7**(4):414

[31] Iakhiaev AV, Nalian A, Koenig K. Thrombin-thrombomodulin inhibits prourokinase-mediated pleural

mesothelial cell-dependent fibrinolysis. Thrombosis Research. 2007;**120**(5):715

[32] Miserocchi G, Pistolesi M, Miniati M, Bellina CR, Negrini D, Giuntini C. Pleural liquid pressure gradients and intrapleural distribution of injected bolus. Journal of Applied Physiology: Respiratory, Environmental and Exercise Physiology. 1984;**56**(2):526

[33] Bhatnagar R, Maskell NA. The modern diagnosis and management of pleural effusions. BMJ. 2015;**351**:h4520. DOI: 10.1136/bmj.h4520

[34] Tschopp JM, Bintcliffe O, Astoul P, Canalis E, Driesen P, Janssen J, Krasnik M, Maskell N, Van Schil P, Tonia T, Waller DA, Marquette CH, Cardillo G. ERS task force statement: Diagnosis and treatment of primary spontaneous pneumothorax. European Respiratory Journal. 2015;**46**(2):321–335. DOI: 10.1183/09031936.00219214

[35] Negrini D, Mukenge S, Del Fabbro M, et al. Distribution of diaphragmatic lymphatic stomata. Journal of Applied Physiology. 1991;**70**:1544–1549

[36] Grimaldi A, Moriondo A, Sciacca L, et al. Functional arrangement of the rat diaphragmatic initial lymphatic network. American Journal of Physiology-Heart and Circulatory Physiology. 2006;**291**:H876–85

[37] Noppen M, De WM, Li R, Gucht KV, D'Haese J, Gerlo E, Vincken W. Volume and cellular content of normal pleural fluid in humans examined by pleural lavage. American Journal of Respiratory and Critical Care Medicine. 2000;**162** (3 Pt 1):1023

[38] Miserocchi G, Negrini D, Mariani E, Passafaro M. Reabsorption of a saline- or plasma-induced hydrothorax. Journal of Applied Physiology: Respiratory, Environmental and Exercise Physiology. 1983;**54** (6):1574

[39] Negrini D, Ballard ST, Jn B. Contribution of lymphatic myogenic activity and respiratory movements to pleural lymph flow. Journal of Applied Physiology. 1994;**76**(6):2267

[40] Wang PM, Lai-Fook SJ. Upward flow of pleural liquid near lobar margins due to cardiogenic motion. Journal of Applied Physiology. 1985;**73**(6):2314

[41] Light RW. Pleural Diseases Philadelphia. 7th ed. Wolters Kluwer; 2022

[42] Tutor JD. Chylothorax in infants and children. Pediatrics. 2014;**133** (4):722–733. DOI: 10.1542/peds. 2013-2072

[43] McGrath EE, Blades Z, Anderson PB. Chylothorax: Aetiology, diagnosis and therapeutic options. Respiratory Medicine. 2010;**104**(1):1–8. DOI: 10.1016/j.rmed.2009.08.010

[44] Rocha G, Arnet V, Soares P, Gomes AC, Costa S, Guerra P, Casanova J, Azevedo I. Chylothorax in the neonate—A stepwise approach algorithm. Pediatric Pulmonology. 2021;**56**(10):3093–3105. DOI: 10.1002/ppul.25601

[45] Beghetti M, La Scala G, Belli D, Bugmann P, Kalangos A, Le Coultre C. Etiology and management of pediatric chylothorax. The Journal of Pediatrics. 2000;**136**(5):653–658. DOI: 10.1067/mpd.2000.104287

[46] Rocha G, Soares P, Rocha P, Quintas C, Martins T, Proença E.

Chylothorax in the fetus and neonate: Guidelines for treatment. Revista Portuguesa de Pneumologia. 2007;**13** (3):377–381. DOI: 10.1016/S0873-2159 (15)30356-1

[47] Bellini C, Hennekam RC. Non-immune hydrops fetalis: A short review of etiology and pathophysiology. American Journal of Medical Genetics Part A. 2012;**158A**(3):597–605. DOI: 10.1002/ajmg.a.34438

[48] Staats BA, et al. The lipoprotein profile of chylous and nonchylous pleural effusions. Mayo Clinic Proceedings. 1980;**55**:700–704

[49] Chan EH, Russell JL, Williams WG, Van Arsdell GS, Coles JG, McCrindle BW. Postoperative chylothorax after cardiothoracic surgery in children. The Annals of Thoracic Surgery. 2005;**80**(5): 1864–1870. DOI: 10.1016/ j.athoracsur.2005.04.048

[50] Merrigan BA, Winter DC, O'Sullivan GC. Chylothorax. The British Journal of Surgery. 1997;**84**(1):15–20. DOI: 10.1046/j.1365-2168.1997.02654.x

[51] Longaker MT, Laberge JM, Dansereau J, et al. Primary fetal hydrothorax: Natural history and management. Journal of Pediatric Surgery. 1989;**24**(6):573–576. DOI: 10.1016/s0022-3468(89)80509-3

[52] Peranteau WH. Thoracoamniotic shunts for the management of fetal lung lesions and pleural effusions: A single-institution review and predictors of survival in 75 cases. Journal of Pediatric Surgery. 2015;**50**:301–305. DOI: 10.1016/j.jpedsurg.2014.11.019

[53] Carr BD, Sampang L, Church JT, Mon RA, Gadepalli S, Attar MA, Perrone EE. Fetal Intervention for Congenital Chylothorax is Associated with Improved Outcomes in Early Life. Journal of Surgical Research. 2018;**231**:361–365. DOI: 10.101 6/j.jss.2018.05.082

[54] Rocha G. Pleural Effusions in the Neonate Current Opinion in Pulmonary Medicine. 2007;**13**(4):305–311. DOI: 10. 1097/MCP.0b013e3281214459

[55] Alvarez OA, Kjellin I, Zuppan CW. Thoracic Lymphangiomatosis in a Child. Journal of Pediatric Hematology/ Oncology. 2004;**26**(2):136–141. DOI: 10 .1097/00043426-200402000-00018

[56] Etoch SW, Bar-Natan MF, Miller FB, thoracostomy RJDT. Factors related to complications. Archives of Surgery. 1995;**130**(5):521–525. DOI: 10.1001/ archsurg.1995.01430050071012

[57] Ball CG, Kirkpatrick AW, Laupland KB, et al. Incidence, risk factors, and outcomes for occult pneumothoraces in victims of major trauma. The Journal of Trauma. 2005;**59** (4):917–924. DOI: 10.1097/01. ta.0000174663.46453.86

[58] Kuhajda I. Penetrating trauma. Journal of Thoracic Disease. 2014;**6** (Suppl 4):S461–S467. DOI: 10.3978/ j.issn.2072-1439.2014.08.51

[59] Gordon CE, Feller-Kopman D. Pneumothorax following thoracentesis: A systematic review and meta-analysis. Archives of Internal Medicine. 2010;**170** (4):332–339. DOI: 10.1001/ archinternmed.2009.548

[60] Yoon SH, et al. Clinical practice guideline for percutaneous transthoracic needle biopsy. Korean Journal of Radiology. 2021;**22**(7): 1050–1070. DOI: 10.3348/kjr.2020.0137

[61] Mowery NT, et al. Practice management guidelines for management of hemothorax and occult pneumothorax. Journal of Trauma: Injury, Infection & Critical Care. 2011;**70**:510–518

[62] Lichtenstein DA. Lung ultrasound in the critically ill. Annals of Intensive Care. 2014;**4**:1. DOI: 10.1186/2110-5820-4-1

[63] Bushby N, Fitzgerald M, Cameron P, Marasco S, Bystrzycki A, Rosenfeld JV, Bailey M. Prehospital intubation and chest decompression is associated with unexpected survival in major thoracic blunt trauma. Emergency Medicine Australasia. 2005;**17**(5-6):443–449. DOI: 10.1111/j.1742-6723.2005.00775.x

[64] Roberts ME, Rahman NM, Maskell NA, Bibby AC, Blyth KG, Corcoran JP, Edey A, Evison M, de Fonseka D, Hallifax R, Harden S, Lawrie I, Lim E, McCracken DJ, Mercer R, Mishra EK, Nicholson AG, Noorzad F, Opstad KS, Parsonage M, Stanton AE, Walker S; BTS Pleural Guideline Development Group. British Thoracic Society Guideline for pleural disease. Thorax. 2023;**78**(Suppl 3):s1–s42. DOI: 10.1136/thorax-2022-219784

[65] Enderson BL, et al. Tube thoracostomy for occult pneumothorax: A prospective randomized study of its use. The Journal of Trauma: Injury, Infection, and Critical Care. 1993;**35**:726–729

[66] Salamonsen MR, Akc L, ACT N, Bashirzadeh F, Wang WYS, Fielding DIK. Novel use of pleural ultrasound can identify malignant entrapped lung prior to effusion drainage. Chest. 2014;**146**(5):1286–1293. DOI: 10.1378/chest.13-2876

[67] Bryant AS, Minnich DJ, Wei B, Cerfolio RJ. The incidence and management of postoperative chylothorax after pulmonary resection and thoracic mediastinal lymph node dissection. The Annals of Thoracic Surgery. 2014;**98**(1):232–237. DOI: 10.1016/j.athoracsur.2014.03.003

[68] McWilliams A, Gabbay E. Chylothorax occurring 23 years postirradiation. Chest. 2000;**117**(3):921–923. DOI: 10.1378/chest.117.3.921

[69] Nair SK, Petko M, Hayward MP. Aetiology and management of chylothorax in adults. European Journal of Cardio-Thoracic Surgery. 2007;**32**(2):362–369. DOI: 10.1016/j.ejcts.2007.04.024

[70] Light RW. Parapneumonic effusions and empyema. Proceedings of the American Thoracic Society. 2006;**3**(1):75–80

[71] Maskell NA, et al. The bacteriology of pleural infection by genetic and standard methods and its mortality significance. American Journal of Respiratory and Critical Care Medicine. 2006;**174**:817–823

[72] Tan J. Association between BMI and recurrence of primary spontaneous pneumothorax. World Journal of Surgery. 2016. DOI: 10.1007/s00268-016-3848-8

[73] Heffner JE, Huggins JT. Managent of Secondary Spontaneous Pneumothorax: There's Confusion in the Air. Chest. 2004;**125**(4):1190–1192. DOI: 10.1378/chest.125.4.1190

[74] Light RW, Macgregor MI, Luchsinger PC, Wc Jr B. Pleural effusions: The diagnostic separation of transudates and exudates. Annals of Internal Medicine. 1972;**77**(4):507–513

[75] Porcel JM, Light RW. Diagnostic approach to pleural effusion in adults. American Family Physician. 2006;**73** (7):1211–1220

[76] Hooper CE, Lee YC, Maskell NA. Setting up a specialist pleural disease service. Respirology. 2010;**15**(7):1028–1036. DOI: 10.1111/j.1440-1843.2010.018 27.x

[77] Rahman NM, et al. Intrapleural use of tissue plasminogen activator and DNase in pleural infection. New England Journal of Medicine. 2011;**365** (6):518–526. DOI: 10.1056/ NEJMoa1012740

[78] American Thoracic Society. Management of malignant pleural effusions. American Journal of Respiratory and Critical Care Medicine. 2000;**162**(5):1987–2001. DOI: 10.1164/a jrccm.162.5.ats8-00

[79] Malignant Pleural Mesothelioma. NCCN Clinical Practice Guidelines in Oncology Washington National Comprehensive Cancer Network (NCCN). 2021. p. 6

[80] Psallidas I, et al. Malignant pleural effusion: From bench to bedside. European Respiratory Review. 2016;**25** (140):189–198. DOI: 10.1183/16000617. 0019-2016

[81] Morris MF. ACR appropriateness criteria workup of pleural effusion or pleural disease. Journal of the American College of Radiology. 2024;**21**(6, Supplement):S343–S352. DOI: 10.1016/ j.jacr.2024.02.013

[82] MacDuff A, Arnold A, Harvey J; BTS Pleural Disease Guideline Group. Management of spontaneous pneumothorax: British thoracic society pleural Disease Guideline 2010. Thorax. 2010;**65**(Suppl 2):ii18–ii31. DOI: 10.1136/thx.2010.136986

[83] Wahidi MM, et al. Management of malignant pleural effusions: American Thoracic Society/STS/STR clinical practice guideline. American Journal of Respiratory and Critical Care Medicine. 2018;**198**(7):839–849. DOI: 10.1164/rcc m.201807-1415ST

[84] Walker WC, Wright V. "Rheumatoid pleuritis". Annals of the Rheumatic Diseases. 1967;**26**(6): 467–474. DOI: 10.1136/ard.26.6.467

[85] Boylan AM, Sanan DA, Sheppard D, Broaddus VC. Vitronectin enhances internalization of crocidolite asbestos by rabbit pleural mesothelial cells via the integrin alpha v beta 5. Journal of Clinical Investigation. 1995;**96**:1987

Section 2

Non-Malignant Pleural Disorders

Chapter 3

Pleural Thickening: Etiology, Radiologic Assessment, and Surgical Management

Ömer Faruk Sağlam

Abstract

Pleural thickening, defined as an increase in the thickness of the parietal or visceral pleura, encompasses a broad spectrum of benign and malignant etiologies with significant diagnostic and therapeutic implications. Globally, chronic infections such as tuberculosis, empyema, and asbestos-related fibrosis are leading benign causes, while malignant pleural mesothelioma and metastatic involvement constitute the most concerning malignancies. Accurate differentiation is vital due to implications for prognosis and management. This chapter offers a comprehensive overview of pleural thickening, beginning with a detailed exploration of its causes, including infectious, inflammatory, occupational, neoplastic, and drug-related factors. Emphasis is placed on imaging modalities: chest radiography for initial assessment, high-resolution computed tomography (CT) as the diagnostic cornerstone, and the adjunctive roles of MRI, thoracic ultrasound, and PET-CT in characterizing extent and metabolic activity. Imaging features such as nodular thickening, mediastinal involvement, and associated effusions aid in distinguishing malignant processes. Definitive diagnosis often requires histopathologic confirmation via image-guided biopsy or video-assisted thoracoscopic surgery (VATS), supported by immunohistochemistry and molecular diagnostics (e.g., BAP1, p16 FISH). Surgical management varies by etiology: decortication is indicated in benign fibrothorax, while pleurectomy/decortication (P/D) or extrapleural pneumonectomy (EPP) may be utilized in selected mesothelioma cases. Future directions include AI-based radiologic interpretation, radiomics, novel PET tracers, liquid biopsy, and molecular profiling to refine diagnosis and personalize treatment. A multidisciplinary approach involving pulmonologists, radiologists, thoracic surgeons, oncologists, and pathologists is critical to optimize outcomes. This chapter bridges evidence-based strategies and technological innovations for effective management of pleural thickening.

Keywords: pleural diseases, pleural thickening, thoracic surgery, diagnostic imaging, radiomics, pleurectomy

1. Introduction

The pleura, a serous membrane enveloping the lungs and lining the thoracic cavity, plays a crucial role in respiratory mechanics by facilitating smooth lung movement during respiration. Pleural diseases encompass a wide spectrum of conditions, ranging from inflammatory processes and infections to malignant transformations. Among these, pleural thickening represents a critical radiologic and pathologic finding with diverse etiologies, often posing significant diagnostic and therapeutic challenges [1].

Globally, pleural diseases are an important health concern due to the continued prevalence of risk factors such as asbestos exposure and tuberculosis in many regions [2, 3]. For instance, an estimated ~30,000 new mesothelioma cases and ~26,000 deaths occur worldwide annually, reflecting the long-term legacy of occupational asbestos use [3]. At the same time, tuberculous pleurisy remains a common cause of pleural thickening in developing countries, occurring in up to 3–30% of tuberculosis patients and often leaving residual fibrous scars in the pleura [4].

This chapter reviews pleural thickening in depth, outlining its benign and malignant causes, diagnostic imaging techniques (computed tomography [CT], magnetic resonance imaging [MRI], ultrasound), histopathologic evaluation, and current surgical treatments such as decortication and pleurectomy. It emphasizes the importance of accurate differentiation between benign and malignant forms, highlights advances such as artificial intelligence (AI) and molecular diagnostics, and provides evidence-based guidance for clinical decision-making. The content addresses a common diagnostic and therapeutic challenge in pulmonology and thoracic surgery, underscoring the value of a multidisciplinary approach.

2. Etiology of pleural thickening

Pleural thickening, defined as an increase in the thickness of either the parietal or visceral pleura, can arise from a multitude of causes and is broadly categorized into benign and malignant conditions. Understanding the underlying etiology is paramount for accurate diagnosis, prognosis, and appropriate management. The diverse origins of pleural thickening underscore the importance of thorough clinical evaluation, often complemented by advanced imaging and, at times, tissue biopsy [5].

2.1. Benign causes

Benign pleural thickening is far more common than its malignant counterpart and often represents the sequelae of prior inflammation, infection, or trauma. Although generally not life-threatening, it can lead to significant morbidity, including decreased lung expansion, impaired respiratory function, and restrictive lung disease [6]. In many patients, a detailed occupational, environmental, and medical history provides important clues (e.g., prior asbestos exposure, tuberculosis infection, trauma, or surgery), but definitive diagnosis often requires imaging and biopsy correlation.

2.1.1. Inflammatory/infectious

Infections are a leading cause of benign pleural thickening. The inflammatory response to various pathogens can lead to fibrin deposition and subsequent fibrosis of the pleural layers. Empyema, a collection of pus in the pleural space, is a particularly potent cause of significant pleural thickening [1]. Organizing empyema, if inadequately drained, leads to fibroblast-driven collagen deposition and the formation of a dense fibrous pleural peel (fibrothorax) that encases the lung, causing a "trapped lung" and severe restrictive dysfunction [4, 7, 8].

The most common cause of chronic diffuse pleural thickening (DPT) is parapneumonic empyema or complicated pleural infection, where inadequate drainage leads to fibrous peel formation (fibrothorax) that restricts lung expansion [4, 9]. Tuberculous pleurisy remains a significant global cause of pleural disease, often presenting as exudative effusion that can resolve with residual thickening and calcification. Studies have reported that 10–72% of patients develop such sequelae despite standard anti-TB therapy [10]. Other infections, including fungal empyema and chronic hemothorax with organizing clots, can similarly produce a dense fibrous pleural rind as a healing response. In post-infectious cases, pleural thickening is typically diffuse, often associated with calcifications and hemithorax volume loss (trapped lung), features that radiologically favor a benign etiology [4, 9].

2.1.2. Trauma and surgery

Trauma and post-pleural injury syndromes, such as hemothorax or post-surgical pleuritis, are common causes of pleural thickening. Blood in the pleural space triggers inflammation and fibrin deposition; if not fully evacuated, it can organize into a dense fibrous peel, often causing localized thickening that may require surgical decortication to restore lung function [11, 12].

2.1.3. Asbestos-related benign pleural disease

Asbestos exposure is a well-established cause of various pleural abnormalities, including benign pleural thickening. This can manifest in several ways.

Pleural plaques: Pleural plaques are the most common benign manifestation of asbestos exposure, appearing as discrete, circumscribed areas of hyalinized collagen on the parietal pleura, typically along the ribs or diaphragm [2, 13]. They often calcify over time and are usually asymptomatic, serving as a biomarker of prior asbestos inhalation without malignant potential. On imaging, they present as focal pleural thickening and therefore enter the differential diagnosis for pleural thickening; their prevalence has been reported to be 1.5% in CT-based cohort studies and up to 50–60% among heavily exposed individuals [2, 4, 13].

Diffuse pleural thickening (DPT): In contrast to plaques, DPT is a more extensive, often non-calcified fibrotic reaction that primarily affects the visceral pleura and can extend to the parietal pleura, resulting in the fusion of pleural layers [2, 14]. DPT commonly develops following a benign asbestos-related pleural effusion, with epidemiologic data indicating that approximately 5–14% of exposed individuals develop sufficient thickening to obliterate the costophrenic angles on chest radiography [2]. Unlike plaques, DPT can cause significant restrictive lung disease and dyspnea, particularly when widespread and circumferential, owing to chronic inflammation and progressive fibrosis in response to inhaled asbestos fibers.

Benign asbestos pleural effusion (BAPE): BAPE can resolve with residual pleural thickening. It is often the earliest manifestation of asbestos-related pleural disease and can occur several years after exposure.

Benign asbestos-related pleural diseases, including plaques, diffuse thickening, and round atelectasis, warrant evaluation for coexisting asbestosis and mesothelioma. They typically present as bilateral smooth thickening or calcified plaques without invasive features but can mimic tumors on imaging.

2.1.4. Drug-induced pleural thickening

Certain medications can induce pleural reactions, including effusions and subsequent pleural thickening. Historically, methysergide has been associated with retroperitoneal and pleural fibrosis. More recently, drugs such as amiodarone, methotrexate, and some beta-blockers have been implicated in drug-induced pleurisy, which can lead to pleural thickening [15]. The mechanism often involves a hypersensitivity reaction or direct toxicity to the pleura.

2.1.5. Drug-induced pleural thickening

Connective tissue diseases, such as rheumatoid arthritis (RA) and systemic lupus erythematosus (SLE), can cause pleuritis that leads to chronic pleural thickening. Rheumatoid pleurisy, more common in middle-aged men with longstanding seropositive RA, may produce exudative effusions that organize into fibrous scars, sometimes showing granulomas and a characteristic "gritty" pleura on thoracoscopy [16, 17]. Recurrent effusions can cause diffuse thickening and occasional calcification, whereas SLE-related pleuritis may result in similar chronic pleural changes, albeit less frequently.

2.1.6. Other rare causes

Uremic pleuritis: Seen in patients with renal failure, it often resolves with dialysis but can leave residual thickening.

Post-radiation pleuritis: Thoracic radiation therapy is a known iatrogenic cause of localized pleural thickening. Patients treated with radiation for breast cancer, lung cancer, or lymphoma often develop unilateral pleural fibrosis within the irradiated field years later [4].

Spontaneous pneumothorax: Recurrent spontaneous pneumothorax can lead to localized pleural adhesions and thickening due to the inflammatory response to air in the pleural space.

Familial mediterranean fever (FMF): This genetic disorder can cause recurrent episodes of serositis, including pleuritis, which may result in chronic pleural thickening [18].

Benign tumors and tumor-like conditions: Certain benign neoplasms or tumor-like processes can appear as pleural thickening on imaging. The most notable is the solitary fibrous tumor of the pleura (SFTP), a mesenchymal neoplasm previously termed benign pleural fibroma or localized fibrous mesothelioma. Approximately 80% of SFTPs are benign and typically present as well-defined, focal pleural-based masses that may produce an obtuse angle with the chest wall on imaging but do not encase the lung. They are often incidental findings, although larger lesions can cause symptoms such as cough, chest pain, or paraneoplastic syndromes, such as hypertrophic osteoarthropathy or hypoglycemia (Doege–Potter syndrome) [4].

In benign conditions, pleural thickening is usually diffuse and smooth rather than nodular, can be unilateral or bilateral, and often shows signs of volume loss, such as an elevated hemidiaphragm or rib crowding if chronic [4]. Calcifications strongly suggest a benign process, particularly post-tuberculous or old empyema [4, 19]. A history of prior infection or asbestos exposure supports this diagnosis. Recognizing benign thickening helps avoid unnecessary invasive procedures, although a biopsy may still be needed to rule out early malignancy.

2.2. Malignant causes

Malignant pleural thickening is a grave finding that is often indicative of advanced disease. It is crucial to differentiate it from benign causes because of the significant differences in prognosis and management. Pleural thickening is a feature of pleural malignancy [20].

2.2.1. Malignant pleural mesothelioma (MPM)

MPM is the most concerning cause of DPT. It is an aggressive neoplasm strongly linked to asbestos exposure, with approximately 80% of cases having significant exposure and a latency of 30–50 years [1, 3, 4, 21]. Although rare, its incidence remains notable worldwide due to past industrial asbestos use, causing approximately 30,000 new cases annually [3]. MPM typically presents in older adults with diffuse, nodular, circumferential pleural thickening that encases the lung, mediastinum, and diaphragm, often accompanied by a large effusion, chest pain, dyspnea, and weight loss [22]. Pathologically, it spreads diffusely along the pleura, forming a rind, with three subtypes: epithelioid (most common), sarcomatoid, and biphasic. Imaging, especially CT and positron emission tomography (PET-CT), is key for suspicion; features include circumferential nodular thickening >1 cm, mediastinal and diaphragmatic involvement, and possible invasion of adjacent structures. However, early disease can mimic benign fibrosis; therefore, a definitive diagnosis requires biopsy. Other risk factors include prior chest irradiation, chronic tuberculous pleuritis, and rare genetic mutations (e.g., BAP1). The prognosis remains poor, with a median survival of approximately 12–18 months [1, 3, 4].

2.2.2. Metastatic pleural disease

Metastatic pleural involvement is far more common than mesothelioma and is the leading cause of malignant pleural effusions, often presenting with pleural thickening. Common primary cancers include lung, breast, ovarian, and gastrointestinal cancers [23, 24]. Metastatic pleural thickening can be focal or diffuse, nodular, and is typically accompanied by effusion and sometimes lymphadenopathy. Imaging often shows multiple discrete nodules or irregular thickening, unlike the symmetric circumferential rind of mesothelioma. For example, lung adenocarcinoma metastases tend to form discrete pleural implants, whereas breast cancer may cause diffuse thickening with effusion but less uniform visceral pleural involvement. Elevated carcinoembryonic antigen (CEA) levels in pleural fluid or blood favor metastatic adenocarcinoma over mesothelioma, which usually does not raise CEA [24]. Accurate distinction is crucial, as management aligns with the primary cancer and often requires immunohistochemistry (IHC) on biopsy.

2.2.3. Lymphoma

Beyond mesothelioma, the pleura can rarely harbor other primary malignancies. Primary pleural lymphoma, often linked to chronic empyema or pyothorax (pyothorax-associated lymphoma), may present as mass-like thickening, typically in immunocompromised patients. Both Hodgkin and non-Hodgkin lymphomas can involve the pleura, causing effusions and nodular or diffuse thickening, usually requiring biopsy for diagnosis.

Other rare primaries include pleural sarcomas (e.g., angiosarcoma, synovial sarcoma), diffuse pleural spread of thymoma or germ cell tumors (sometimes called "drop metastases"), and pleural epithelioid hemangioendothelioma – a vascular tumor of intermediate malignancy. These entities are uncommon and are diagnosed only after excluding more frequent causes with histopathologic confirmation.

In summary, malignant pleural thickening is most often due to diffuse malignant mesothelioma or metastatic carcinomatosis. Radiologically, features favoring a malignant cause include nodular pleural thickening exceeding 1 cm in thickness, circumferential involvement of the hemithorax, involvement of the mediastinal pleural surface, and extension into the fissures or chest wall [4, 21]. The presence of a concomitant pleural effusion is common in malignancy (although benign effusions can coexist with inflammation as well). Because clinical and radiographic findings can overlap between benign and malignant causes, tissue biopsy is usually required for definitive diagnosis when malignant disease is suspected. The following sections will delve into the imaging characteristics that help differentiate these etiologies and the diagnostic procedures used to obtain tissue for histopathologic evaluation.

3. Radiologic assessment of pleural thickening

Radiologic assessment is fundamental for detecting, characterizing, and differentiating pleural thickening. Imaging helps define the extent, morphology (diffuse vs. focal, smooth vs. nodular, calcified vs. non-calcified), and features suggesting benign or malignant causes. It also guides biopsy by pinpointing accessible abnormal pleura and is essential for staging in malignancy. Multiple modalities provide complementary information, and the choice depends on clinical suspicion and disease extent. The following sections outline the key imaging techniques and their roles in distinguishing benign from malignant pleural thickening [20].

3.1. Imaging modalities

3.1.1. Chest radiography (X-ray)

Chest radiography is often the first imaging modality for detecting pleural disease but has limited sensitivity for assessing pleural thickening [1, 9, 20]. Diffuse thickening may appear on a posteroanterior (PA) radiograph as a smooth, continuous pleural density extending over at least 25% of the chest wall, with possible blunting or obliteration of the costophrenic angle that does not shift with patient position, indicating fibrosis rather than fluid [4, 25]. Focal calcified plaques can be seen as curvilinear opacities along the ribs, diaphragm, or lateral chest wall, while an apical cap is common with aging; however, thickening over ~2 cm should raise suspicion for prior tuberculosis or malignancy.

A classic radiographic clue is the "extrapleural sign," where a pleural-based lesion creates an opacity with smooth, tapered margins forming obtuse angles with the chest wall, suggesting a pleural or extrapleural origin rather than a parenchymal mass. Both benign and malignant processes can produce this sign; for example, a chronic calcified empyema or a pleural tumor [4]. However, chest radiography often underestimates the true extent of thickening and cannot reliably distinguish benign from malignant causes. Small nodules (<5 mm) may be entirely missed, and diffuse thickening from mesothelioma may mimic fibrotic changes from old TB empyema. Therefore, significant pleural abnormalities on radiography should prompt further cross-sectional imaging for definitive characterization [20, 21].

3.1.2. Computed tomography (CT)

Chest CT is the gold-standard imaging modality for the detailed assessment of pleural thickening [22]. It provides high-resolution cross-sectional images that allow precise evaluation of pleural thickness, extent, morphology, and relationship with adjacent structures [22]. Key features assessed on CT include the following [4, 19, 21, 22, 26–28]:

Location and extent: CT differentiates between localized and diffuse thickening and identifies involvement of the parietal, visceral, diaphragmatic, and mediastinal pleura. The normal pleura is only approximately 1–2 mm thick, and any visible thickening suggests pathology.

Morphology: CT distinguishes smooth, uniform thickening (more typical of benign fibrosis) from nodular or irregular thickening, which is concerning for malignancy. Nodules >1 cm, circumferential encasement of the lung, and mediastinal pleural involvement strongly suggest malignancy, particularly mesothelioma.

Calcification: The pattern of calcification helps identify benign causes, such as asbestos plaques or old empyema. Chronic benign thickening often shows associated pleural calcification.

Associated findings: CT can identify associated pleural effusions, parenchymal lung abnormalities, lymphadenopathy, and chest wall invasion, all of which are crucial for differential diagnosis.

Benign versus malignant patterns: Malignant pleural disease (e.g., mesothelioma) typically shows nodular or irregular thickening >1 cm, circumferential pleural rind encasing the lung, mediastinal pleural surface involvement, fissure and chest wall invasion, and enhancement after IV contrast.

Benign thickening usually appears smooth and uniform, less than ~10 mm thick except in localized areas, spares the mediastinal pleura or shows mild involvement, displays volume loss, rib crowding, diaphragmatic elevation, and may exhibit the "extrapleural fat sign"—hypertrophy of extrapleural fat adjacent to chronic fibrosis. Quantitative criteria such as continuous thickening >5 cm in length, >8 cm vertically, and >3 mm thick can support a benign diagnosis but are not absolute.

Role in biopsy and staging: CT is essential for planning image-guided pleural biopsies, targeting areas of maximum nodularity or thickness. Non-contrast CT can detect subtle pleural changes in high-risk patients (e.g., asbestos exposure), whereas contrast-enhanced CT better characterizes suspicious lesions and enhancement patterns. For mesothelioma, CT helps to stage local tumor spread (T stage) and assess nodal involvement.

Limitations: CT may underestimate chest wall or diaphragmatic invasion due to limited soft tissue contrast and may miss small metastases. There is also inter-observer variability in interpreting subtle pleural changes, reinforcing the need for correlation between clinical history and other modalities.

3.1.3. Magnetic resonance imaging (MRI)

MRI offers excellent soft tissue contrast and is increasingly utilized in the evaluation of pleural thickening, particularly when differentiating between benign and malignant etiologies, assessing chest wall invasion, or evaluating diaphragmatic involvement [28]. MRI can provide functional information through diffusion-weighted imaging (DWI) and dynamic contrast-enhanced (DCE) sequences, which can help distinguish between active tumors and fibrous tissue. Although not routinely used as a first-line imaging modality for pleural thickening, MRI is valuable in specific scenarios, such as in patients with contraindications to iodinated contrast or when a detailed assessment of soft tissue invasion is required.

3.1.4. Ultrasound

Thoracic ultrasound is a readily available, non-invasive, and radiation-free imaging modality that is highly valuable for the assessment of pleural diseases [20]. It is particularly useful for the following reasons:

Detection of pleural effusions: Ultrasound can detect small pleural effusions, even those not visible on chest X-ray, and characterize their nature (e.g., anechoic, septated, complex).

Guidance for procedures: It is indispensable for guiding thoracentesis and pleural biopsy, minimizing the risks of complications.

Assessment of pleural thickening: Ultrasound can visualize pleural thickening and assess its vascularity using Doppler. Although less precise than CT for detailed morphologic characterization, it can identify nodularities or masses on the pleural surface and differentiate between fluid and solid components [29].

3.1.5. Positron emission tomography (PET-CT)

PET-CT, typically performed with 18F–fluorodeoxyglucose (FDG), provides functional metabolic information that complements anatomical imaging in the evaluation of pleural thickening [4, 21, 30].

Differentiating benign versus malignant: Malignant pleural lesions show increased glucose metabolism and, therefore, high FDG uptake (The maximum standardized uptake value [SUVmax]), whereas benign fibrous thickening generally has low or absent uptake. Qualitative and quantitative PET analysis can help distinguish tumors from scar tissue; for example, SUVmax values above 2.0–2.5 may suggest malignancy. However, false positives can occur because of inflammation (e.g., post-talc pleurodesis), and some early-stage mesotheliomas may have low uptake, risking false negatives.

Staging: PET-CT is highly valuable in staging MPM and metastatic pleural disease by detecting nodal and distant metastases, which is essential for treatment planning and surgical decision-making. Pre-operative workups are routinely recommended to avoid futile surgeries in patients with unresectable disease.

Guiding biopsy: Areas of high metabolic activity can guide targeted biopsies, improving diagnostic yield by sampling the most suspicious sites.

Monitoring treatment response: Changes in FDG uptake can reflect the metabolic response earlier than visible size changes on CT, aiding in therapy monitoring.

Limitations: While PET/CT enhances diagnostic confidence, it cannot alone confirm or exclude malignancy due to overlapping uptake in inflammation and cancer. Findings must always be interpreted in the context of other imaging, clinical history, and histopathology [21, 31].

3.2. Differentiating benign versus malignant pleural thickening

The ability to distinguish between benign and malignant pleural thickening is critical because of the vastly different prognoses and management strategies. Although no single imaging feature is pathognomonic, a combination of findings across different modalities can help narrow the differential diagnosis. Radiologists use qualitative visual assessment to distinguish between benign and malignant disease once pleural thickening is identified [21].

3.2.1. Imaging features suggestive of malignancy

Nodularity: The presence of discrete nodules or irregular, lumpy thickening within the pleura is a strong indicator of malignancy, particularly in the context of mesothelioma or metastatic disease [1].

Circumferential thickening: Involvement of the entire circumference of the pleura encasing the lung is highly suggestive of MPM [22]. DPT is defined as thickening of the pleura (>5 mm) with a combined area of involvement [4].

Mediastinal pleural involvement: Thickening of the mediastinal pleura, especially if nodular, is a concerning sign of malignancy.

Parietal and visceral pleural involvement: Malignant processes often involve both layers of the pleura, leading to a rind-like appearance.

Associated pleural effusion: While benign conditions can cause effusions, a large, rapidly reaccumulating, or hemorrhagic effusion in conjunction with pleural thickening raises suspicion for malignancy.

Chest wall or diaphragmatic invasion: Direct extension of pleural thickening into the chest wall, diaphragm, or mediastinal structures is a definitive sign of malignancy.

Contralateral pleural involvement: While less common, bilateral malignant pleural thickening can occur with metastatic disease.

High FDG uptake on PET-CT: As discussed, increased metabolic activity on PET-CT is a strong indicator of malignancy.

3.2.2. Imaging features suggestive of benignity

Smooth, non-nodular thickening: Benign thickening often appears smooth and uniform, without discrete nodules.

Localized thickening: Benign processes tend to cause localized thickening, such as apical caps or focal areas related to prior inflammation.

Calcification: The presence of calcification, particularly in the form of discrete pleural plaques or diffuse calcification from old empyema or TB, is characteristic of a benign etiology [13]. However, calcification rarely occurs in mesothelioma.

Stable appearance over time: Benign pleural thickening typically remains stable or shows slow progression over long periods, whereas malignant thickening often demonstrates rapid progression.

Absence of associated mass or lymphadenopathy: The lack of a discrete pleural mass or regional lymph node involvement favors a benign process.

Radiologic findings can strongly suggest the cause of pleural thickening but are not definitive. Histopathologic evaluation of pleural tissue remains the gold standard for differentiating benign from malignant processes and for diagnosing specific conditions such as tuberculosis or distinct tumor types. Therefore, pleural biopsy, which provides tissue for histologic and sometimes microbiologic analysis, is essential when imaging and clinical features raise the suspicion of malignancy or when the etiology is unclear. This section outlines biopsy techniques, characteristic histopathologic features of major causes, and the role of ancillary tests such as IHC and molecular markers in diagnosis.

3.3. Role of imaging in biopsy guidance

Given the overlap in imaging features between benign and malignant pleural thickening, tissue diagnosis is often required for a definitive diagnosis. Imaging plays a crucial role in guiding biopsy procedures to ensure adequate tissue acquisition and minimize complications. Ultrasound and CT are commonly used to guide percutaneous pleural biopsies, allowing real-time visualization of the needle trajectory and targeting of suspicious areas, particularly nodular or metabolically active regions identified on PET/CT. Thoracoscopy video-assisted thoracoscopic surgery (VATS) also relies on imaging for pre-procedural planning and intraoperative guidance to select appropriate biopsy sites.

4. Histopathologic features and diagnosis

Once pleural tissue is obtained, pathologic evaluation focuses on distinguishing among three main possibilities: benign pleuritis or fibrosis, diffuse malignant mesothelioma, and metastatic malignancy (or other rare primary tumors). Accurate diagnosis relies on histologic features and the use of special stains and ancillary tests.

4.1. Benign pleural thickening (fibrosis)

Benign pleural thickening from prior inflammation shows dense collagenous fibrosis, typically pauci-cellular with scattered lymphocytes or plasma cells, and possible calcifications.

Tuberculous pleuritis: Features granulomatous inflammation with epithelioid histiocytes, Langhans giant cells, and central caseation necrosis; acid-fast bacilli may be rare, so cultures or **polymerase chain reaction** (PCR) assist in diagnosis.

Rheumatoid pleuritis: Shows fibrin deposits and rheumatoid granulomas with central necrosis and palisading histiocytes.

Key clue: Benign fibrosis does not invade the adjacent fat or muscle. Reactive mesothelial cells may form surface layers but lack invasive growth and significant atypia. Limited samples may still yield an "atypical mesothelial proliferation" diagnosis, prompting further biopsy or close follow-up.

4.2. Malignant mesothelioma

Definitive diagnosis requires evidence of invasive, neoplastic mesothelial cells.

Subtypes:

Epithelioid: Uniform cuboidal to polygonal cells forming tubules, papillae, or sheets; resembles adenocarcinoma but lacks mucin production.

Sarcomatoid: Spindle cell sheets resembling fibrous tissue; more aggressive and harder to differentiate morphologically.

Biphasic: Contains both epithelioid and sarcomatoid areas.

Immunohistochemistry (IHC): Mesothelioma typically expresses calretinin, Wilms's Tumor 1 (WT1), cytokeratin 5/6 (CK5/6), and Podoplanin (D2-40), and is negative for lung carcinoma markers such as carcinoembryonic antigen (CEA), thyroid transcription factor 1 (TTF-1), and monoclonal antibody clone 31 (MOC-31) [32]. The standard practice is to use ≥2 positive mesothelial markers and ≥2 negative carcinoma markers for confirmation.

Ancillary markers: Loss of BRCA1 Associated Protein 1 (BAP1) nuclear staining supports mesothelioma (observed in approximately 50–67% of cases); cyclin-dependent kinase inhibitor 2A (CDKN2A [p16]) deletion by fluorescence in situ hybridization (FISH) further supports the diagnosis in challenging cases [33].

Consensus: Accurate diagnosis integrates morphology, immunohistochemistry (IHC), and molecular tests, with referral to specialized centers if needed.

4.3. Metastatic pleural malignancies

Carcinomas in pleural biopsies often represent metastases or direct extension from another primary tumor.

Lung adenocarcinoma: TTF-1+, Napsin A+, CEA+; shows glandular structures and mucin production.

Breast carcinoma: GATA3+, Estrogen Receptors/Progesterone Receptors (ER/PR)+, and Gross Cystic Disease Fluid Protein-15 (GCDFP-15)+.

Squamous carcinoma: p40+, CK5/6+; distinguished from mesothelioma by keratinization and the lack of WT1.

Extrapulmonary cancers: for example, ovarian carcinoma, may be WT1+ (like mesothelioma) but also paired box gene 8 (PAX8)+, which mesothelioma lacks. Each case requires a tailored IHC panel to confirm the primary source.

Lymphoma: Sheets of atypical lymphocytes suggest lymphoma, confirmed by immunophenotyping or flow cytometry. Pyothorax-associated lymphomas (e.g., Epstein-Barr virus [EBV]-related diffuse large B-cell lymphoma) are rare but have been recognized.

In summary, histopathology, IHC, and ancillary molecular tests are critical for distinguishing benign pleuritis, mesothelioma, and metastatic disease, ensuring accurate diagnosis and appropriate treatment planning.

A multidisciplinary approach that combines imaging, history, and pathology is essential for accurate diagnosis and management. For example, asbestos-related fibrosis with an inconclusive biopsy may require close follow-up for mesothelioma risk, while confirmed benign pleurisy after empyema can help avoid overtreatment. Histopathology also clarifies the exact tumor type, guiding decisions between surgery and systemic therapy.

5. Surgical management of pleural thickening

Surgical management of pleural thickening ranges from observation for asymptomatic benign conditions to complex multimodal surgery for malignancies such as mesothelioma. Indications and techniques vary significantly depending on the etiology, extent of disease, patient comorbidities, and treatment goals. Surgery can be diagnostic, therapeutic, or both, and must be integrated with medical therapies and careful patient selection to optimize outcomes [34].

5.1. Indications for surgical intervention

5.1.1. Diagnostic purposes

When imaging and less invasive procedures (e.g., thoracentesis and closed pleural biopsy) fail to yield a definitive diagnosis, surgical biopsy becomes necessary. VATS is the gold standard for obtaining adequate pleural tissue for histopathologic examination, particularly in cases of suspected malignancy (e.g., mesothelioma, metastatic disease) or chronic inflammatory conditions where a specific diagnosis is elusive [35]. VATS allows for direct visualization of the pleura and targeted biopsies of suspicious areas and often provides a larger tissue sample than percutaneous methods.

5.1.2. Therapeutic purposes

Therapeutic indications for the surgical management of pleural thickening primarily aim to alleviate symptoms, restore lung function, or remove diseased tissue.

Symptomatic relief: Significant pleural thickening, especially DPT, fibrothorax, or organized empyema, can cause severe dyspnea due to restrictive lung physiology. Surgical decortication can free the trapped lung, allowing it to re-expand and improve respiratory mechanics (e.g., vital capacity <50–70% predicted) [6–8]. Decortication removes the inelastic fibrous peel, allowing full lung re-expansion and symptomatic relief.

Lung re-expansion: In cases of trapped lung secondary to organized hemothorax or empyema, the fibrous peel prevents the lung from re-expanding. Decortication is performed to remove the peel and facilitate full lung expansion [8].

Tumor debulking/resection: In MPM, surgery aims for macroscopic complete resection (MCR) of visible tumors as part of a multimodality treatment plan that includes chemotherapy and/or radiotherapy [36]. Surgery alone is not curative because of microscopic spread; however, cytoreduction can improve local control, symptom relief, and possibly survival in selected patients. Pleurectomy/decortication (P/D) and extrapleural pneumonectomy (EPP) are the principal surgical options, with P/D now preferred in many centers due to lung preservation and lower morbidity [19, 20].

Management of recurrent pleural effusions: While not directly treating thickening, pleurodesis or placement of indwelling pleural catheters (IPCs) controls recurrent effusions often associated with pleural malignancy or chronic exudates. Pleurodesis induces pleural adhesion to obliterate the pleural space and prevent fluid reaccumulation [37]. IPCs allow outpatient drainage, improving the quality of life in patients unfit for surgery [33].

5.2. Surgical techniques

Several surgical techniques are employed in the management of pleural thickening, ranging from minimally invasive approaches to extensive resection.

5.2.1. Thoracentesis and pleural drainage (brief mention for context)

While not strictly surgical management of thickening, thoracentesis (diagnostic or therapeutic) and chest tube drainage are often the initial steps in managing pleural effusions that may lead to or be associated with pleural thickening. They are crucial for fluid analysis and temporary symptom relief but do not address the underlying thickening directly [15].

5.2.2. Video-assisted thoracoscopic surgery (VATS)

VATS has revolutionized thoracic surgery, offering a minimally invasive approach for both diagnostic and therapeutic interventions for pleural diseases. For pleural thickening, VATS is widely used for:

Diagnostic biopsy: As mentioned, VATS provides excellent visualization and allows for multiple targeted biopsies, significantly increasing diagnostic yield compared to blind or image-guided percutaneous biopsies [38].

Pleurodesis: Chemical or mechanical pleurodesis can be performed via VATS to prevent the recurrence of pleural effusions, particularly in malignant cases. This involves inducing inflammation and adhesion between the parietal and visceral pleura [39].

Decortication/debridement: In early or localized cases of organized empyema or hemothorax, VATS can be used for debridement and removal of fibrinous material, facilitating lung re-expansion [12].

Advantages of VATS include smaller incisions, reduced pain, shorter hospital stays, and faster recovery compared to open thoracotomy.

5.2.3. Decortication

Decortication involves the surgical removal of the dense fibrous pleural peel that restricts lung expansion and is indicated for symptomatic trapped lung in chronic empyema, organized hemothorax, or fibrothorax. It can be performed via VATS for early-stage disease or open thoracotomy for dense, mature peels [7, 40, 41]. Outcomes are excellent: lung function typically improves by approximately 10–15% in forced expiratory volume in the first second/forced vital capacity (FEV_1/FVC, Tiffeneau-Pinelli index), with >90% achieving full re-expansion in well-selected patients. Mortality is low (<2% in modern series) [7, 8, 41].

5.2.4. Pleurectomy

Pleurectomy involves the surgical removal of the pleura. It can be partial or complete, involving either the parietal pleura (lining the chest wall) or the visceral pleura (covering the lung), or both. This is often performed in the context of the following:

Recurrent pleural effusions: Parietal pleurectomy can be performed to achieve permanent pleurodesis and prevent fluid reaccumulation, particularly in benign recurrent effusions or when chemical pleurodesis has failed.

Malignant pleural mesothelioma (MPM): Pleurectomy is a key component of the surgical management of MPM [36]. Parietal pleurectomy involves the removal of the parietal pleura, while visceral pleurectomy involves stripping the visceral pleura from the lung surface. In many cases of MPM, extended P/D is performed, which involves the removal of both parietal and visceral pleura, along with any gross tumor, from the lung, diaphragm, and pericardium, while preserving the lung [42]. This procedure aims to achieve complete macroscopic resection of the tumor.

5.2.5. Extrapleural pneumonectomy (EPP) and pleurectomy/decortication (P/D) in malignant pleural mesothelioma (MPM)

For patients with MPM, two main surgical approaches are considered for curative intent [36]:

Extrapleural Pneumonectomy (EPP): This is a radical procedure involving en bloc removal of the ipsilateral lung, parietal and visceral pleura, ipsilateral diaphragm, and pericardium. EPP aims for complete microscopic resection and is associated with significant morbidity and mortality. It is typically reserved for highly selected patients with early-stage disease, good performance status, and no evidence of nodal or distant metastases [43].

Pleurectomy/decortication (P/D): As described above, P/D is a lung-sparing procedure that involves the extensive removal of all macroscopic tumors from the pleura, diaphragm, and pericardium, while preserving the lung. P/D is generally associated with lower morbidity and mortality than EPP and is increasingly favored, especially for patients who may not tolerate EPP or have more advanced disease where lung preservation is desirable. The goal of P/D is MCR, which has been shown to improve survival in selected patients [40]. In one study, P/D had a median 30-day mortality of 2.2% and a median overall survival of 21 months [44].

Both EPP and P/D are typically part of a multimodal treatment strategy that includes chemotherapy and/or radiation therapy.

5.2.6. Other surgical considerations

Pleurodesis: This procedure induces adhesion between the parietal and visceral pleura to obliterate the pleural space and prevent fluid reaccumulation. It can be achieved chemically (e.g., talc slurry, doxycycline) or mechanically (e.g., pleural abrasion during VATS). It is commonly used for recurrent malignant pleural effusions [39].

Indwelling pleural catheters (IPCs): For patients with recurrent symptomatic pleural effusions who are not candidates for pleurodesis or more invasive surgery, IPCs offer a palliative option for outpatient drainage and symptom control. While not a surgical treatment for thickening, they manage the associated effusion [34].

5.3. Post-operative management and complications

Post-operative management following pleural surgery is critical for optimal outcomes. It typically involves pain control, chest tube management, respiratory physiotherapy, and close monitoring of complications. Potential complications include prolonged air leak, infection (empyema), hemorrhage, atelectasis, pneumonia, and, in the case of EPP, acute respiratory distress syndrome (ARDS) or right heart failure. Empyemas are associated with parietal pleural thickening in 86% of cases and pleural enhancement in 96% of patients [45]. Careful patient selection, meticulous surgical techniques, and comprehensive post-operative care are essential to minimize these risks and optimize recovery.

6. Emerging concepts and future directions

The landscape of pleural disease diagnosis and management is evolving rapidly. Several emerging concepts show promise in improving how clinicians differentiate and manage the diverse causes of pleural thickening. Key innovations include the use of AI and radiomics in advanced imaging analysis, alongside molecular diagnostics and biomarkers that enable earlier or more precise detection of malignant pleural processes.

6.1. Artificial intelligence and radiomics in pleural imaging

Radiomics involves extracting large sets of quantitative features from imaging (CT, MRI, and PET) that can reveal subtle disease characteristics beyond what the eye can detect. Studies demonstrate that radiomic models can match expert radiologists in distinguishing benign from malignant pleural thickening and can support diagnostic decisions for less experienced readers [21]. For instance, radiomics applied to PET/CT scans in mesothelioma has shown prognostic value in predicting progression-free survival [21].

Machine learning (ML) and deep learning (DL) build on radiomics by automating pattern recognition directly from raw images. In mesothelioma, DL models have been developed to segment tumors and measure volumes, thereby improving the accuracy and reproducibility of disease burden assessments [46, 47]. AI models can also aid in early classification; a multicenter study by Li et al. (2022) achieved 95%

accuracy in differentiating mesothelioma from metastatic pleural disease using CT-based ML features [24].

Despite these advances, AI models face challenges with generalizability owing to variability in scanners and protocols. Additionally, their "black box" nature can limit clinician trust. Nevertheless, AI holds clear potential to complement traditional imaging, for example, flagging subtle thickening on a routine scan or providing a malignancy risk score that prompts timely biopsy.

Emerging PET tracers represent another area of innovation. While FDG remains the standard, research into novel tracers (e.g., mesothelin- or integrin-targeted agents) may further refine the differentiation of scar tissue from active tumors when combined with AI-assisted interpretation.

6.2. Molecular diagnostics and biomarkers

Molecular tools aim to enable earlier detection and better confirmation of malignancy, especially for mesothelioma.

Circulating biomarkers:

Soluble mesothelin-related peptide (SMRP) is the only FDA-approved biomarker for mesothelioma diagnosis and monitoring, with good specificity but moderate sensitivity [48]. Other candidates—fibulin-3, osteopontin, High mobility group box 1 protein (HMGB1) – and microRNAs (e.g., MicroRNA [miR]-126) show promise, although they require further validation [48, 49].

Liquid biopsy:

The detection of circulating tumor DNA (ctDNA) with mesothelioma-specific mutations (such as BAP1 and Neurofibromatosis type II [NF2]) is under investigation. Although ctDNA levels are often low, advances in sequencing may eventually allow for monitoring and earlier relapse detection.

Molecular pathology:

Markers such as BAP1 loss and p16 (CDKN2A) deletion by FISH are now standard ancillary tests to distinguish mesothelioma from benign reactive processes [50]. Gene expression profiling and PCR-based panels could enhance accuracy in ambiguous biopsies.

Genomics and personalized therapy:

Deep sequencing has mapped common mesothelioma mutations, opening the door to trials of targeted or synthetic lethal therapies, especially in BAP1-deficient tumors [51]. Immunotherapy (e.g., nivolumab + ipilimumab) is now a standard systemic option [52]. Predictive molecular signatures for treatment response are being developed, moving toward personalized care.

AI in pathology:

Early studies show that ML algorithms can aid pathologists by differentiating mesothelioma from adenocarcinoma on digitized slides, potentially enhancing diagnostic accuracy in centers with limited expertise.

7. Conclusion

Pleural thickening is a frequent but diagnostically challenging finding in thoracic practice, encompassing a spectrum from benign post-inflammatory fibrosis to aggressive malignancies such as mesothelioma. This chapter outlines the diverse etiologies, radiologic strategies for assessment, the critical role of histopathology, and tailored management approaches, including surgery.

Imaging, especially high-resolution CT, remains the cornerstone for detecting and characterizing pleural thickening, with MRI, ultrasound, and PET/CT offering valuable complementary insights. The integration of AI-driven analysis and functional imaging holds promise to reduce diagnostic uncertainty and reliance on invasive procedures.

Surgical management must be individualized.

Decortication remains definitive for benign trapped lung (e.g., post-empyema fibrothorax).

For MPM, extended P/D has largely supplanted EPP owing to lower morbidity and similar survival in carefully selected patients.

Multimodal therapy, combining surgery, systemic treatments, and, in some cases, radiation, is essential, and recent trials emphasize careful patient selection.

Future directions include refining radiologic and molecular tools to detect malignancy earlier, improving staging, and tailoring therapies based on individual tumor profiles. Immunotherapy and targeted therapies continue to expand the options for patients historically faced with poor prognoses.

Finally, the importance of a multidisciplinary approach cannot be overstated. Collaborative care involving pulmonologists, radiologists, thoracic surgeons, oncologists, and pathologists ensures accurate diagnosis and optimal management, whether that means simple surveillance of stable benign plaques or aggressive multimodal therapy for early mesothelioma.

By applying evidence-based principles and embracing technologic advancements, clinicians can improve the outcomes of patients with pleural thickening worldwide.

Acknowledgments

The author acknowledges the use of ChatGPT-4 (OpenAI) and Paperpal (Editage) for language editing and polishing of the manuscript. These tools were used solely to improve the clarity, coherence, and academic tone of the text. The author retains full responsibility for the content and interpretation of the manuscript.

Author details

Ömer Faruk Sağlam
Thoracic Surgery, Tokat State Hospital, Tokat, Turkey

*Address all correspondence to: mrfrksglm@gmail.com

References

[1] Lee GM, Walker CM. Pleural thickening: Detection, characterization, and differential diagnosis. Seminars in Roentgenology. 2023;**58**:399–410. DOI: 10.1053/j.ro.2023.06.001.

[2] Ferreiro L, Toubes ME, Rodríguez-Núñez N, Valdés L. Asbestos and benign pleural diseases: A narrative review. Breathe. 2025; **21**. 240236. DOI: 10.1183/20734735.0236-2024.

[3] Han Y, Zhang T, Chen H, Yang X. Global magnitude and temporal trend of mesothelioma burden along with the contribution of occupational asbestos exposure in 204 countries and territories from 1990 to 2019: Results from the Global Burden of disease study 2019. Critical Reviews in Oncology/Hematology. 2022; **179**. 103821. DOI: 10.1016/j.critrevonc.2022.103821.

[4] Sureka B, Thukral BB, Mittal MK, Mittal A, Sinha M. Radiological review of pleural tumors. Indian Journal of Radiology and Imaging. 2013;**23**:313–320. DOI: 10.4103/0971-3026.125577.

[5] Naeger DM. Diseases of the pleura and chest wall. In Hodler J, K-hra RJE, editors. Diseases of the Chest, Heart and Vascular system 2025-2028. Cham: Springer, 2025:39–48. DOI: 10.1007/978-3-031-83872-9_4.

[6] Krishna R, Antoine MH, Alahmadi MH, et al. Pleural effusion. [Updated 2024 Aug 31]. StatPearls [Internet]; Treasure Island (FL): StatPearls Publishing; 2025 Jan. Available from: https://www.ncbi.nlm.nih.gov/books/NBK448189/

[7] Özer KB, Tükel M, Özdemir A, Cesur EE, Demirhan R. The effects of pleural decortication on respiratory functions of the patients having pleural empyemas. Southern Clinics of Istanbul Eurasia. 2018. DOI: 10.14744/scie.2018.85866

[8] Kumar A, Anand SLD. Lung Decortication [Updated 2022 November 7]. In: StatPearls [Internet]. Treasure Island (FL): StatPearls Publishing; 2025 Jan. Available from: https://www.ncbi.nlm.nih.gov/books/NBK564375/

[9] Saito A, Hakamata Y, Yamada Y, Sunohara M, Tarui M, Murano Y, Mitani A, Tanaka K, Nagase T, Yanagimoto S. Pleural thickening on screening chest X-rays: A single institutional study. Respiratory Research. 2019;**20**:138

[10] Zhu Y, Gao Y-H, Zou J-N, Xi E-P. Beware of pleural thickening and calcification: An enlightenment from a case of Tuberculous Pleurisy. Risk Management and Healthcare Policy. 2021;**14**:1551–1554. DOI: 10.2147/RMHP.S303614.

[11] Qureshi NR, and Gleeson FV. Pleural Thickening, Benign Diffuse. In Encyclopedia of Diagnostic Imaging. Berlin, Heidelberg: Springer Berlin Heidelberg, 2008: 1507–1508. DOI: 10.1007/978-3-540-35280-8_1972. Baert, AL eds

[12] Redden MD, Chin TY, van Driel ML. Surgical versus non-surgical management for pleural empyema. Cochrane Database of Systematic Reviews. 2017;**2017**. DOI: 10.1002/14651858.CD010651.pub2.

[13] Araki T, Yanagawa M, Sun FJ, Dupuis J, Nishino M, Yamada Y, Washko GR, Christiani DC, Tomiyama

N, O'Connor GT, Hunninghake GM, Hatabu H. Pleural abnormalities in the Framingham Heart Study: Prevalence and CT image features. Occupational & Environmental Medicine. 2017;**74**: 756–761

[14] Miles SE, Sandrini A, Johnson AR, Yates DH. Clinical consequences of asbestos-related diffuse pleural thickening: A review. Journal of Occupational Medicine and Toxicology. 2008;**3**:20. DOI: 10.1186/1745-6673-3-20.

[15] Karkhanis V, Joshi J. Pleural effusion: Diagnosis, treatment, and management. Open Access Emergency Medicine. 2012;31. doi:10.2147/OAEM. S29942

[16] Huggins JT, Sahn SA. Causes and management of pleural fibrosis. Respirology. 2004;**9**:441–447. DOI: 10.1111/j.1440-1843.2004.00630.x.

[17] Shaw M, Collins BF, Ho LA, Raghu G. Rheumatoid arthritis-associated lung disease. European Respiratory Review. 2015;**24**:1–16. DOI: 10.1183/09059180.00008014.

[18] Katsenos S, Mermigkis C, Psathakis K, Tsintiris K, Polychronopoulos V, Panagou P, Ritis K, Light RW, et al. Unilateral Lymphocytic Pleuritis as a manifestation of familial mediterranean fever. Chest. 2008;**133**:999–1001

[19] Weerakkody Y, Campos A, Silverstone L. Malignant pleural disease. Radiopaedia.org. 2010. DOI: 10.53347/rID-8730

[20] Hassan M, Touman AA, Grabczak EM, Skaarup SH, Faber K, Blyth KG, Pochepnia S. Imaging of pleural disease. Breathe. 2024;**20**: 230172. 230172. DOI: 10.1183/20734735.0172-2023

[21] Romei C, Fanni SC, Volpi F, Milazzo A, D'Amore CA, Colligiani L, Neri E, De Liperi A, Stella GM, Bortolotto C. New updates of the imaging role in diagnosis, staging, and response treatment of malignant Pleural Mesothelioma. Cancers (Basel). 2021;**13**:4377

[22] Gabelloni M, Faggioni L, Brunese MC, Picone C, Fusco R, Aquaro GD, Cioni D, Neri E, Gandolfo N, Giovagnoni A, Granata V. An overview on multimodal imaging for the diagnostic workup of pleural mesothelioma. Japanese Journal of Radiology. 2024;**42**:16–27

[23] Yamada A, Taiji R, Nishimoto Y, Itoh T, Marugami A, Yamauchi S. Pictorial review of pleural disease: Multimodality imaging and differential diagnosis. RadioGraphics. 2024:44. DOI: 10.1148/rg.230079.

[24] Li Y, Cai B, Wang B, Lv Y, He W, Xie X, Hou D. Differentiating malignant pleural mesothelioma and metastatic pleural disease based on a machine learning model with primary CT signs: A multicentre study. Heliyon. 2022;**8**:e11383

[25] Hallifax RJ, Talwar A, Wrightson JM, Edey A, Gleeson FV. State-of-the-art: Radiological investigation of pleural disease. Respiratory Medicine. 2017;**124**:88–99. DOI: 10.1016/j. rmed.2017.02.013.

[26] Evans AL, Gleeson FV. Radiology in pleural disease: State of the art. Respirology. 2004;**9**:300–312. DOI: 10.1111/j.1440-1843.2004.00599.x.

[27] Katz SI, Straus CM, Roshkovan L, Blyth KG, Frauenfelder T, Gill RR, Lalezari F, Erasmus J, Nowak AK, Gerbaudo VH, Francis RJ, Armato SG, et al. Considerations for imaging of

Malignant Pleural Mesothelioma: A consensus statement from the International Mesothelioma interest group. Journal of Thoracic Oncology. 2023;**18**:278–298

[28] Lauk O, Patella M, Neuer T, Battilana B, Frauenfelder T, Nguyen-Kim TDL, Weder W, Caviezel C, Hillinger S, Inci I, Opitz I, et al. Implementing CT tumor volume and CT pleural thickness into future staging systems for malignant pleural mesothelioma. Cancer Imaging. 2021;**21**:48

[29] Kamel KM, El-Hinnawy YH. Role of transthoracic ultrasound in differentiation of the causes of pleural thickening. Egyptian Journal of Bronchology. 2018;**12**:260–265. DOI: 10.4103/ejb.ejb_109_17.

[30] Kramer H, Pieterman RM, Slebos D-J, Timens W, Vaalburg W, Koëter GH, Groen HJM. PET for the evaluation of pleural thickening observed on CT. Journal of Nuclear Medicine : Official Publication, Society of Nuclear Medicine. 2004;**45**:995–998

[31] Weerakkody Y, Luong D, Kang O. Tuberculous pleuritis. Radiopaedia.org; 2020. DOI: 10.53347/rID-78816

[32] Raparia K, Schneider F, Roden A, Dacic S, Baker TP Protocol for the examination of specimens from patients with diffuse Pleural Mesothelioma. College of American Pathologists 2024. https://documents.cap.org/protocols/PleuraPericard_5.0.0.0.REL.CAPCP.pdf [accessed June 1, 2025]

[33] Louw A, Lee YCG, Acott N, Creaney J, van Vliet C, Chai SM. Diagnostic utility of BAP1 for malignant pleural mesothelioma in pleural fluid specimens with atypical morphology. Cytopathology. 2022;**33**:84–92. DOI: 10.1111/cyt.13015.

[34] Roberts ME, Rahman NM, Maskell NA, Bibby AC, Blyth KG, Corcoran JP, Edey A, Evison M, de Fonseka D, Hallifax R, Harden S, Lawrie I, Lim E, McCracken D, Mercer R, Mishra EK, Nicholson AG, Noorzad F, Opstad KS. British Thoracic society guideline for pleural disease. Thorax. 2023;**78**:1143–1156

[35] Dhanasopon AP, Blasberg JD, Mase VJ. Surgical management of Pneumothorax and pleural space disease. Surgical Clinics of North America. 2022;**102**:413–427. DOI: 10.1016/j.suc.2022.03.001.

[36] Lapidot M, Sattler M. The Role of Surgery in Pleural Mesothelioma. Cancers (Basel). 2024;**16**:1719. DOI: 10.3390/cancers16091719.

[37] Bhatnagar R, Corcoran JP, Maldonado F, Feller-Kopman D, Janssen J, Astoul P. Advanced medical interventions in pleural disease. European Respiratory Review. 2016;**25**:199–213

[38] Ciuche A, Nistor C, Pantile D, Prof Horvat T. Minimally invasive surgical treatment of malignant pleural effusions. Maedica (Bucur). 2011;**6**:262–267

[39] Ali M, Sharma S, Surani S. Pleurodesis. 2025 Jan 19. StatPearls [Internet]. Treasure Island (FL): StatPearls Publishing; 2025 Jan

[40] Abraham SV, Chikkahonnaiah P. Change in Pulmonary function following decortication for chronic Pleural Empyema. Turkish Thoracic Journal. 2020;**21**:27–31. DOI: 10.3390/cancers13174377.

[41] Boffa DJ, Mason DP, Su JW, Murthy SC, Feng J, McNeill AM, et al. Decortication after Lung transplantation. The Annals of Thoracic Surgery. 2008;**85**:1039–1043

[42] Paajanen J, Jaklitsch MT, Bueno R. Contemporary issues in the surgical management of pleural mesothelioma. Journal of Surgical Oncology. 2023;**127**:343–354. DOI: 10.1002/jso.27152.

[43] Scarci M, Abah U, Solli P, Page A, Waller D, van Schil P, Melfi F, Schmid RA, Athanassiadi K, Sousa Uva M, Cardillo G, et al. EACTS expert consensus statement for surgical management of pleural empyema. European Journal of Cardio-Thoracic Surgery. 2015;**48**:642–653

[44] Elsayed HH, Abdel-Gayed M. Survival and mortality after extrapleural pneumonectomy versus pleurectomy/decortication for malignant pleural mesothelioma: A systematic review. The Cardiothoracic Surgeon. 2024;**32**:25. DOI: 10.1186/s43057-024-00144-y.

[45] Shen KR, Bribriesco A, Crabtree T, Denlinger C, Eby J, Eiken P. The American Association for Thoracic Surgery consensus guidelines for the management of empyema. The Journal of Thoracic and Cardiovascular Surgery. 2017;**153**:e129–46

[46] Gudmundsson E, Straus C, Li F, Kindler H, Armato S. P1.06-04 deep learning-based segmentation of Mesothelioma on CT scans: Application to patient scans exhibiting pleural effusion. Journal of Thoracic Oncology. 2019;14:S478. doi:10.1016/j.jtho.2019.08.991

[47] Kidd AC, Anderson O, Cowell GW, Weir AJ, Voisey JP, Evison M, Tsim S, Goatman KA, Blyth KG, et al. Fully automated volumetric measurement of malignant pleural mesothelioma by deep learning AI: Validation and comparison with modified RECIST response criteria. Thorax. 2022;**77**:1251–1259

[48] Pass HI, Alimi M, Carbone M, Yang H, Goparaju CM. Mesothelioma Biomarkers: A review highlighting contributions from the early detection research network. Cancer Epidemiology Biomarkers and Prevention. 2020;**29**:2524–2540. DOI: 10.1158/1055-9965.EPI-20-0083.

[49] Wang -J-J, Yan L. Serum diagnostic markers for malignant pleural mesothelioma: A narrative review. Translational Cancer Research. 2022;**11**:4434–4440. DOI: 10.21037/tcr-22-2873.

[50] Husain AN, Chapel DB, Attanoos R, Beasley MB, Brcic L, Butnor K, Chirieac LR, Churg A, Dacic S, Galateau-Salle F, Hiroshima K, Hung YP, Klebe S, Krausz T, Khoor A, Litzky L, Marchevsky A, Nabeshima K, Nicholson AG. Guidelines for pathologic diagnosis of Mesothelioma: 2023 update of the consensus statement from the International Mesothelioma Interest Group. Archives of Pathology and Laboratory Medicine. 2024;**148**:1251–1271

[51] Schunselaar LM, Zwart W, Baas P. Targeting BAP1: A new paradigm for mesothelioma. Lung Cancer: Targets Ther. 2017;**109**:145–146. DOI: 10.1016/j.lungcan.2017.03.005.

[52] Cardillo G, Waller D, Tenconi S, Di Noia V, Ricciardi S. Malignant Pleural Mesothelioma: A 2025 update. Journal of Clinical Medicine. 2025;**14**:1004. DOI: 10.3390/jcm14031004.

Chapter 4

Benign Asbestos-Related Disorders of the Pleura

Richard L. Kradin

Abstract

Asbestos is a generic term for six naturally occurring fibrous silicates that were used extensively in the twentieth century, primarily for their insulating properties. Following their introduction into the workplace, it was noted that a variety of benign and malignant diseases were caused by asbestos. These included a diffuse scarring disorder of the lungs termed "asbestosis," as well as both lung cancer [1] and mesothelioma [2]. Although benign asbestos-related disorders of the pleura rarely cause symptoms or are life-threatening, they are markers of asbestos exposure that can be detected radiographically. They can enter into the differential diagnosis with malignancy, and as such, it is important to be cognizant of their features and how they are diagnosed.

Keywords: asbestos, pleura, effusion, plaques, mesothelioma, fibrosis, chrysotile, amphibole, talc

1. Introduction

Asbestos is a generic term for six naturally occurring fibrous mineral silicates (chrysotile, amosite, crocidolite, anthophyllite, tremolite, actinolite), used extensively during the twentieth century for their ability to be woven into textiles with insulating properties. Unfortunately, asbestos can cause a variety of life-threatening disorders, including diffuse pulmonary fibrosis (asbestosis) and cancer (lung carcinoma and mesothelioma). Asbestosis was recognized in the 1920s as a progressive, diffuse interstitial scarring disorder of the lung capable of leading to pulmonary restriction, hypoxemia, cor pulmonale, and death. Later in the twentieth century, it was established that asbestos was also a cause of lung cancer and malignant mesothelioma, the latter being a highly lethal malignancy of the pleura. However, asbestos can also cause several benign disorders of the pleura that can present diagnostic challenges [1] as shown in **Table 1**.

1.1 Pleural anatomy

The normal pleura is invisible to the naked eye and only several cells thick. It consists of a fibrous matrix lined by a single layer of cuboidal mesothelial cells with no basement membrane. The visceral pleura lines the surfaces of both lungs and is

Benign asbestos-related pleural effusion (BAPE)
Benign asbestos-related pleural plaques (BAPP)
Benign asbestos-related diffuse pleural fibrosis (DPF)
Rounded atelectasis (RA)

Table 1.
Benign asbestos-related disorders.

separated from the underlying lung by an ill-defined elastic lamina. The parietal pleura is continuous with the visceral pleura and lines the surfaces of the chest wall, mediastinum, and diaphragmatic leaflets [2]. Mesothelial cells also line the pericardium and abdominal viscera.

Pleural mesothelial cells normally secrete small quantities of non-viscid fluid that act to reduce surface friction resulting from the periodic expansion and contraction of the lungs within the thoracic cavity. They exhibit elongated microvilli with surfaces capable of reabsorbing excess fluid, thereby maintaining fluid homeostasis within the pleural cavity. When inflamed, mesothelial cells both proliferate and increase their level of fluid secretion out of proportion to their ability to absorb it. This results in pleural effusions that may be detectable by physical examination and radiographic imaging. Inflammation may cause symptoms, including pleuritic pain and dyspnea, due to restriction of the underlying lung. The inflamed pleura exhibits microvascular injury that leads to fibrinous exudates and the accumulation of inflammatory cells in the pleura and the surrounding effusion. When inflammation is chronic, the pleural matrix becomes fibrotic, with adhesions to the surface of the adjacent lung that can result in pulmonary restriction.

Under normal conditions, the pleura is a "privileged site," largely protected from toxic elements in the external environment. However, the pleura contains lymphatic channels that communicate with the periphery of the adjacent lung, thereby serving as a channel for particles in the ambient air to reach the pleura. A superficial plexus of lymphatic vessels courses within the visceral pleura and over the convex surface of the lung to drain to lymph nodes in the pulmonary hilum [3].

Greater than 95% of inhaled asbestos fibers are either expelled from the lungs during normal ventilation or swallowed. However, the small percentage of fibers that deposit in the lungs following occupational exposure to asbestos may represent millions of fibers, as a single gram of asbestos has been estimated to contain in excess of a trillion (10^{12}) microscopic fibers [4].

The fate of asbestos fibers in the lung varies with fiber type. Chrysotile, also known as white or serpentine asbestos, has a short half-life in the lung, measured in days to weeks [5]. Pulmonary macrophages can ingest these fibers and leach their magnesium content within the acidic environment of their lysosomes, leading to their further breakdown and disappearance. In contrast, needle-like fibers of amphibole asbestos have a high aspect ratio (length:width ≥3.0) and exhibit half-lives in the lung, often measured in years to decades. In the lung, a small percentage of both chrysotile and amphibole fibers become encrusted with iron and, as a result, can be detected by light microscopy. However, ferruginized "asbestos bodies" are rarely observed in the pleura [6].

A fraction of the chrysotile and amphibole fibers that deposit in the peripheral lung is rapidly translocated to the pleura via peripheral lymphatics, where they can redeposit in the pleura and cause disease. Although all types of asbestos fibers can persist in the pleura, chrysotile asbestos has been the dominant fiber type observed in the pleura in patients with mesothelioma [7]. After depositing in the pleura, asbestos fibers can induce inflammatory cells to generate toxic free radicals and cytokines that contribute both to fibrosis and the malignant transformation of mesothelial cells [8].

2. Benign asbestos-related pleural effusion (BAPE)

Benign pleural effusion attributable to asbestos exposure occurs in approximately 20% of individuals occupationally exposed to asbestos [9] as shown in **Table 2**. First reported in 1964 by Eisenstadt, the demographics of BAPE have varied across case series [9]. Most cases occur in men and are unilateral, with a slight left-sided predominance [10]. Initially thought to occur within ten years of the first exposure to asbestos, some cases have been reported with latencies measured in decades [11]. In one study, the median age for the development of BAPE was 61.8 years, with a median latency of 24 years following exposure [12].

There is no correlation between the intensity of exposure to asbestos and the development of BAPE. The usual clinical course is spontaneous resolution within six months. However, BAPE effusions can recur, raising concern for underlying malignancy, although BAPE has not been demonstrated to be an independent risk factor for malignant mesothelioma.

While the pathogenesis of BAPE is uncertain, proposed pathways include (1) direct injury to pleural tissues by asbestos fibers within the adjacent lung that penetrate into the adjacent pleura, (2) induction of inflammation by those asbestos fibers that deposit in the pleura, and (3) hypersensitivity reactions to fibers in the pleura. The latter are often associated with eosinophilia in the pleural fluid. The pleural fluid in BAPE is exudative, may be bloody, and shows lymphocytic predominance. The fluid shows no specific serological features that distinguish it reliably from other causes of exudative effusions [9]. When the index of suspicion for malignancy is high, a pleural biopsy is indicated. When biopsied, the pleura in BAPE shows non-specific reactive fibrinous pleuritis and fibrosis (see **Figure 1**).

Suggested diagnostic criteria include (1) a history of previous asbestos exposure, (2) pleural effusion confirmed by radiology, (3) the exclusion of other causes (such as parapneumonic effusion, empyema, malignancy, pulmonary embolism, pancreatitis,

Approximately 20% of individuals occupationally exposed to asbestos
More common in men
Usually unilateral
May occur early or late after exposure
Subset may be hypersensitivity reactions
Usually resolves spontaneously within six months
Must exclude other benign causes and malignancies

Table 2.
Benign asbestos pleural effusion (BAPE).

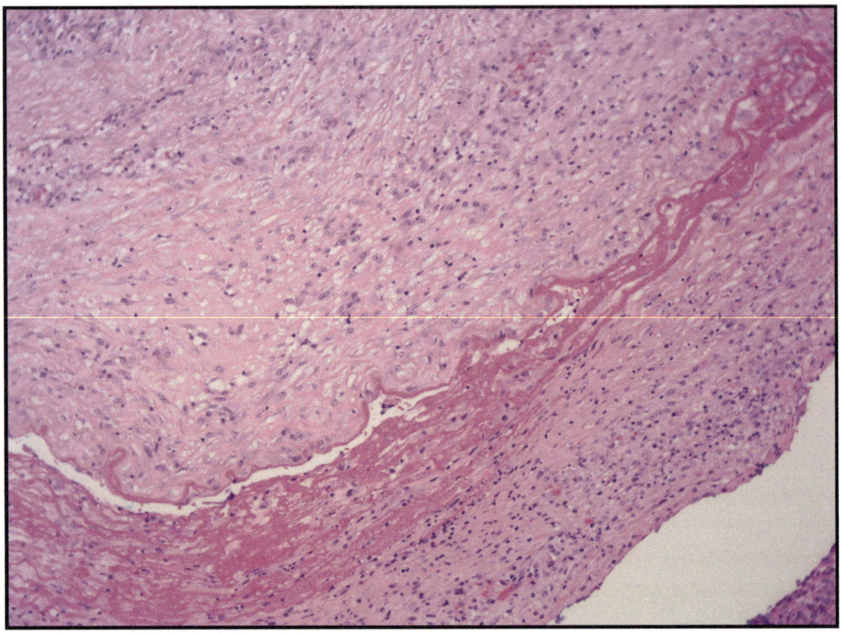

Figure 1.
The pathology of BAPE shows organizing fibrinous pleuritis.

and connective tissue disease), and (4) no evidence of a malignant tumor within three years of diagnosis, with emphasis on the exclusion of other causes.

Kato et al. found that the prevalence of pleural plaques was significantly higher in patients with BAPE compared to pleural effusions caused by other factors, and "low-level" pleural irregularities (<1 cm) were also more frequent [13].

3. Benign asbestos pleural plaques (hyaline pleural plaques)

Pleural plaques occur in approximately 60% of individuals with previous occupational exposure to asbestos [9] (see **Table 3**). They have been detected in 2%–12% of all patients undergoing autopsy in urban areas. Pleural plaques have been observed as early as six years following exposure but may take decades to develop [14]. Chest CT scans are more sensitive than conventional chest radiographs at detecting pleural plaques (see **Figure 2(a)**); however, autopsy remains the gold standard for their detection.

The amount of asbestos required to produce pleural plaques is uncertain, and no threshold of exposure for their development has been demonstrated. However, heavy exposure to asbestos is not required to produce plaques. Plaques have developed in individuals exposed directly and occupationally to asbestos, bystanders to work involving asbestos-containing materials, and individuals exposed to asbestos deposited on the clothing and person of workers, most often by those laundering the clothing of workers [15]. Although, in most cases, pleural plaques have developed in individuals exposed to amosite asbestos, exposure to chrysotile alone can also cause pleural plaques [16].

Seen in approximately 50% of occupationally exposed individuals
85% bilateral
Along the lateral chest wall and diaphragmatic leaflets
May be seen in the pericardium and spleen
May occur within several years of exposure or later
Tend to calcify
Majority are detected by CT scan, but autopsy is the gold standard
Characteristic pauci-cellular hyalinized collagen by histology
Objective markers of asbestos exposure
Can be seen following talc exposure
Largely asymptomatic

Table 3.
Benign asbestos-related pleural plaque (BAPP).

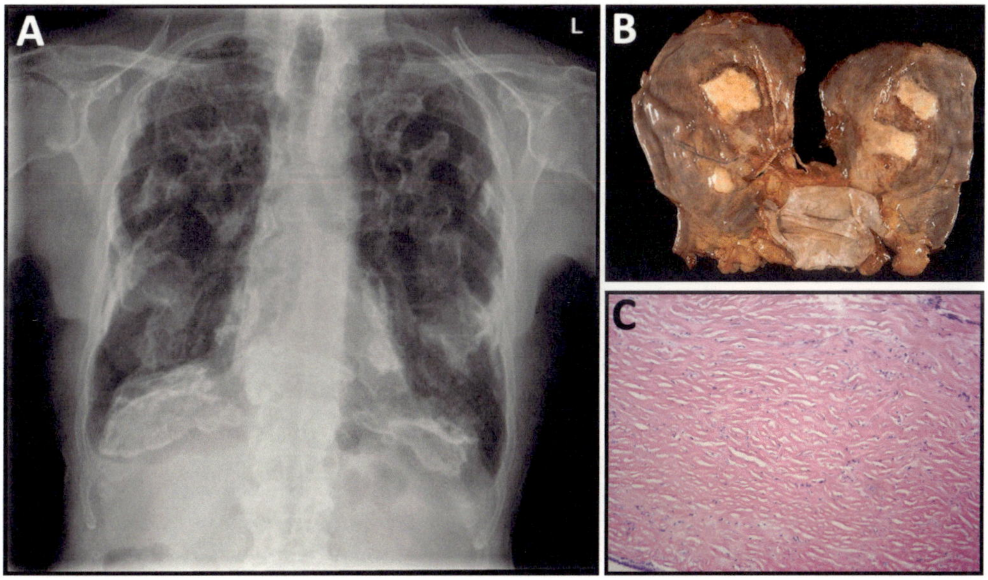

Figure 2.
(a) Chest radiograph shows multiple en face *calcified pleural plaques. (b) Calcified pleural plaques mimicking "candlewax drippings" along diaphragmatic leaflets in an autopsy specimen. (c) Histology shows characteristic paucicellular hyalinized collagenous plaque.*

Individuals exposed to talc, including remote talc pleurodesis and, less often, cosmetic talc, have developed calcified plaques indistinguishable in their histologic and radiographic appearance from those seen following exposure to asbestos [17]. As deposits of talc are often contaminated with asbestos, including chrysotile, tremolite, anthophyllite, and actinolite, it is likely that the plaques seen following talc exposure are also caused by asbestos [18].

At autopsy, plaques are recognizable as discrete raised areas along the pleural surfaces and are bilateral in approximately 85% of cases [9]. Asbestos-related pleural plaques tend to develop along the posterolateral surfaces of the parietal pleura adjacent to the fifth to eighth thoracic ribs but can be seen along any of the pleural surfaces, including the visceral pleura, as well as on mesothelial-lined surfaces of the pericardium, aortic adventitia, and splenic capsule [19]. They are most characteristically seen along the thoracic surfaces of the diaphragmatic leaflets. Over time, fibrous plaques can absorb circulating calcium, and when heavily calcified, they resemble white to yellow "candle droppings" of wax at autopsy (see **Figure 2(b)**).

3.1 Pathogenesis

Asbestos promotes the generation of free radicals and profibrotic cytokines, including IL-1, IL-6, and TGF-beta, from macrophages. This results in the deposition of collagen within the pleura. The pathological appearance of benign asbestos-related pleural plaques includes localized pleural thickening that is histopathologically characteristic, as it is (1) pauci-inflamed and (2) exhibits a basket-weave appearance of hyalinized type I collagen. The histology is sufficiently unique under the light microscope to be distinguishable from other reactive fibrotic changes of the pleura and is essentially diagnostic of previous exposure to asbestos (see **Figure 2(c)**).

3.2 Physiology

The vast majority of individuals with radiographically detected pleural plaques are asymptomatic, and pulmonary function testing generally shows no abnormality in the absence of concomitant pulmonary asbestosis. However, when plaques are extensive, they may produce a restrictive defect.

4. Diffuse pleural fibrosis (DPF)

Asbestos causes clinically detectable diffuse pleural thickening in approximately 5% of individuals occupationally exposed to asbestos and can lead to fibrothorax and pulmonary restriction [9] (see **Table 4**). In the past, this disorder was referred to as *plaque en cuirasse*, as the fibrotic pleura encasing the underlying lung, when calcified, resembles the armor of a medieval knight. Symptoms of dyspnea, especially with exercise, and a sensation of chest "tightness" may be reported. Severe cases have been associated with CO_2 retention and respiratory failure [20].

Approximately 5% of individuals occupationally exposed to asbestos
Usually unilateral
May be symptomatic
Pulmonary restriction
Treatment is decortication, if necessary

Table 4.
Diffuse asbestos-related pleural fibrosis (DPF).

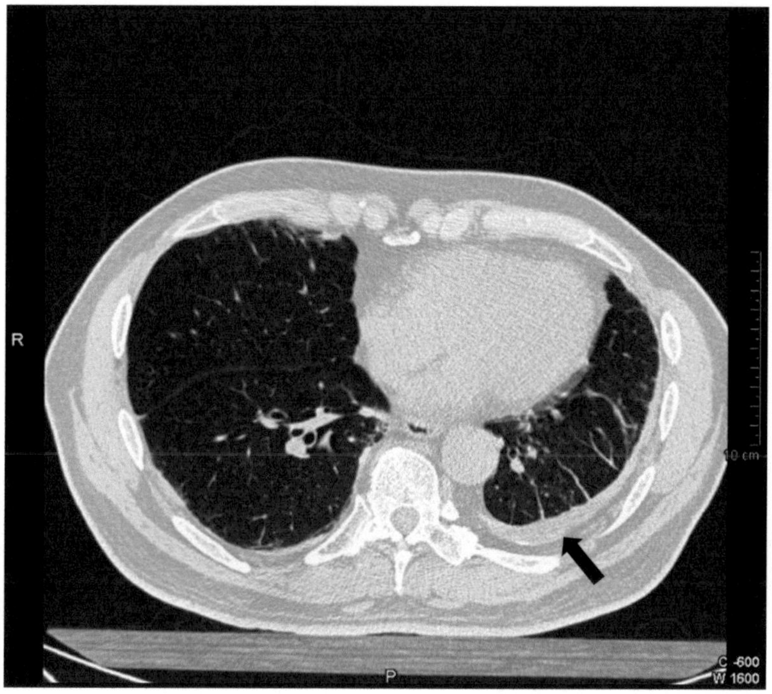

Figure 3.
CT scan reveals diffuse pleural fibrosis (arrow).

Chest radiographs can reveal pleural thickening, but chest CT or MRI are more sensitive for establishing the diagnosis and can be useful for distinguishing between DPF and extrapleural fat [21] (see **Figure 3**).

The treatment, when required, is surgical decortication to release the entrapped underlying lung. However, when underlying asbestosis is present, efforts at pulmonary re-expansion are often unsuccessful [22].

5. Rounded atelectasis

This disorder was described by Blesovsky in 1966 as “folded lung” but is now widely referred to as “rounded atelectasis” (see **Table 5**). More than half of patients with rounded atelectasis report a history of exposure to asbestos [11]. Areas of rounded atelectasis can be solitary or multiple and are often located in the middle and lower lung zones. Rounded atelectasis can be mistaken for pulmonary malignancy and lead to invasive biopsy or lung resection when its characteristic radiographic features are not recognized.

The pathophysiology of rounded atelectasis is thought to be due to adhesions between a parietal pleural plaque and the underlying visceral pleura, leading to folding of the underlying lung. Alternatively, it has been suggested that rounded atelectasis may result from pleurogenic fibrosis, that is, the extension of pleural fibrosis into a subjacent fissure that limits the local expansion of the underlying lung, resulting in progressive atelectasis of the lung. Pathologically, one observes what

Frequency uncertain
50% of individuals with RA report exposure to asbestos
"Pseudotumor" noted radiographically
Associated with localized pleural thickening
May be multiple
Characteristic "comet sign" on CT scan
Must be distinguished from malignancy

Table 5.
Rounded atelectasis (RA).

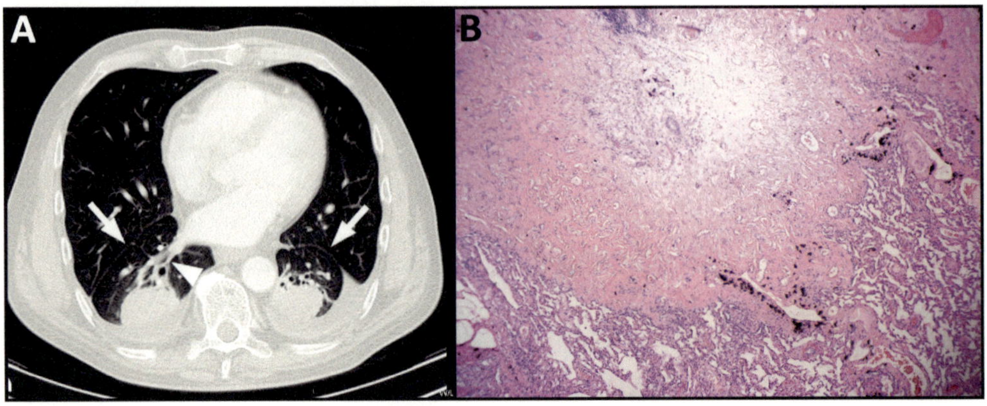

Figure 4.
(a) CT scan shows multiple areas of rounded atelectasis with the "comet sign." (b) Histology of rounded atelectasis showing a pseudotumor of collapsed fibrotic alveolar septa.

appears to be fibrotic alveolated lung collapsed into a ball-like structure subjacent to an area of adhered visceral and parietal plaques (see **Figure 4**).

The CT radiographic appearance of this disorder is essentially pathognomonic. One observes a mass associated with what has been referred to as a "comet's tail" that courses toward the hilum [23] (see **Figure 4**). The periphery of the mass is subjacent to a pleural plaque. The pseudotumor is denser at its center, and one can often identify an airway leading into it. This appearance virtually excludes pulmonary malignancy, and an occupational history along with the association of calcified pleural plaques signals the underlying cause. In the vast majority of cases, no treatment is required. In the rare situation where areas of rounded atelectasis are large and/or multiple, the loss of functional lung parenchyma may be sufficient to cause symptoms [24].

6. Mesothelioma *in situ*

Although not a benign disorder of the pleura *per se,* the *in situ* growth of mesothelioma can occur years before the development of frankly invasive malignancy and can be confused with BAPE.

The existence of an *in situ* phase of malignant mesothelioma had been postulated for decades but was difficult to prove. However, with the advent of tumor genetic analysis, it is now possible to identify mesothelial cells that harbor genetic mutations seen only in malignant cells and not in benign mesothelial proliferations. These include bi-allelic *BAP-1* mutations (a member of the BAP1 family) and *CDKN2A* (p16) deletions. The loss of nuclear expression of *BAP-1* is commonly present as an acquired somatic mutation (~50% of epithelioid mesotheliomas) but can rarely occur as a germline (non-acquired) defect in families. Bi-allelic deletion of *CDKN2A* is present in 60%–80% of tumors [25].

Distinguishing benign from malignant mesothelial cells via analysis in cytology and tissue biopsy specimens currently allows for distinguishing mesothelioma *in situ* from benign proliferative reactions. Recent studies suggest that the application of immunostains for MTAP (methylthioadenosine phosphorylase) can serve as a reliable marker for the expression of *CDKN2A/p16*. Loss of MTAP expression by immunostaining strongly suggests malignant transformation [26]. In a similar vein, loss of nuclear BAP-1 protein expression by immunostaining correlates with the loss of the *BAP-1* gene and is a reliable marker of neoplastic transformation.

In 2018, Churg et al. described ten patients with mesothelioma *in situ,* which they defined as a single layer of atypical surface mesothelial cells showing loss of BAP1 nuclear immunostaining, with no evidence of tumor by imaging or invasive mesothelioma for at least one year [27] (see **Figure 5**). Nine were pleural mesotheliomas, and most were biopsied for repeated effusions of uncertain etiology. In two patients, mesothelioma *in situ* was an incidental finding in lungs resected for a concomitant pulmonary carcinoma. *CDKN2A* was deleted by FISH (fluorescence *in situ* hybridization)analysis in one of eight cases.

Invasive malignant mesothelioma subsequently developed in seven patients 12 to 92 months following the diagnosis of *in situ* mesothelial neoplasia, but there was no evidence of invasive mesothelioma in three patients after 12, 57, and 120 months of follow-up. The authors concluded that mesothelioma *in situ* is associated with a high risk of developing invasive mesothelioma over a protracted period.

The most recent WHO classification of thoracic malignancies includes malignant mesothelioma *in situ* as a distinct diagnostic entity. According to the WHO criteria,

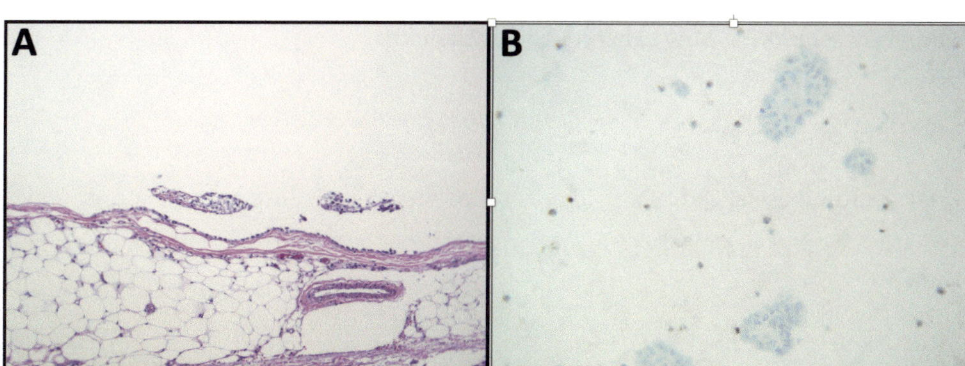

Figure 5.
(a) Pleural biopsy reveals a single layer of plump mesothelial cells. (b) Nests of mesothelial cells from effusion reveal a lack of nuclear immunostaining for BAP-1, characteristic of mesothelioma in situ.

"mesothelioma is clinically suspected in patients presenting with non-resolving pleural effusions in the setting of heavy asbestos exposure, with or without pleural plaques, and in patients with familial predisposition. The diagnosis is based on a combination of clinical, imaging, and pathological features." However, it should be noted that this differs from the standard definition of most *in situ* malignancies, which are ascertained exclusively by histologic evidence of malignancy without tissue invasion. The confident diagnosis of mesothelioma *in situ* requires "extensive" thoracoscopic sampling of the tumor, and small biopsies or cytological sampling are insufficient to exclude invasive malignant mesothelioma.

To date, only a small number of cases of malignant mesothelioma *in situ* have been reported. These have been predominantly in the pleura and in men in their seventh decade. However, demographics do not distinguish *in situ* mesothelioma from invasive malignancy. Klebe et al. noted that an international survey of 34 pulmonary pathologists with an interest in malignant mesothelioma diagnosis exhibited inconsistencies regarding how the diagnosis of *in situ* mesothelioma was established, despite published guidelines [28]. Diagnosing the *in situ* phase of most malignancies generally triggers surgical excision with a high cure rate. However, as patients are often elderly with significant co-morbidities, malignant mesothelioma *in situ* may not be amenable to this approach. Since the subsequent timing of the development of invasive disease is uncertain, how best to approach a diagnosis of mesothelioma *in situ* remains unclear. Nevertheless, it must be distinguished from recurrent BAPE.

7. Conclusion

Although largely benign with respect to their clinical course, the non-malignant disorders of the pleura attributable to asbestos can present clinical challenges. In the case of pleural plaques, their presence on chest radiographic imaging is sufficiently characteristic to state confidently that a patient has previously been exposed to asbestos, a point that often comes up in medical–legal cases where exposure to asbestos has been claimed. As the malignant disorders related to asbestos can require decades to develop, demonstrating a benign asbestos-related disorder should alert the clinician that an individual should be followed closely in the future for evidence of either pulmonary asbestosis, lung cancer, or mesothelioma.

Conflicts of interest

Dr. Kradin has served as a paid consultant in asbestos litigation.

Author details

Richard L. Kradin
Honorary Pathologist and Associate Physician, Massachusetts General Hospital, Emeritus in Medicine and Pathology, Harvard Medical School, Boston, USA

*Address all correspondence to: richardkradin@gmail.com

References

[1] Kradin RL. Understanding Pulmonary Pathology. New York: Academic Press; 2017.

[2] Sevin CM, Light RW. Microscopic anatomy of the pleura. Thoracic Surgery Clinics. 2011;**21**(2):173–5,vii.

[3] Burke HE. The lymphatics which drain the potential space between the visceral and the parietal pleura. American Review of Tuberculosis. 1959;**79**(1):52–65.

[4] Visona SD, et al. Evaluation of deposition and clearance of asbestos (detected by SEM-EDS) in lungs of deceased subjects environmentally and/ or occupationally exposed in Broni (Pavia, Northern Italy). Frontiers in Public Health. 2021;**9**:678040.

[5] Coin PG, Roggli VL, Brody AR. Deposition, clearance, and translocation of chrysotile asbestos from peripheral and central regions of the rat lung. Environmental Research. 1992;**58**(1): 97–116.

[6] Churg A, Warnock ML. Analysis of the cores of ferruginous (asbestos) bodies from the general population. I. Patients with and without lung cancer. Laboratory Investigation; A Journal of Technical Methods and Pathology. 1977;**37**(3):280–286.

[7] Suzuki Y, Kohyama N. Translocation of inhaled asbestos fibers from the lung to other tissues. American Journal of Industrial Medicine. 1991;**19** (6):701–704.

[8] Pociask DA, Sime PJ, Brody AR. Asbestos-derived reactive oxygen species activate TGF-beta1. Laboratory Investigation. 2004;**84**(8):1013–1023.

[9] Ferreiro L, et al. Asbestos and benign pleural disease. Breathe. 2025;**21**:240236–240240.

[10] Cugell D, Kamp D. Asbestos and the pleura: A review. Chest. 2004;**125**:1103–1117.

[11] Hillerdal G, Ozesmi M. Benign asbestos pleural effusion: 73 exudates in 60 patients. European Journal of Respiratory Diseases. 1987;**71**(2): 113–121.

[12] Fujimoto N, et al. Clinical investigation of benign asbestos pleural effusion. Pulmonary Medicine. 2015;**2015**:416179–416185.

[13] Kato K, et al. Pleural irregularities and mediastinal pleural involvement in early stages of malignant pleural mesothelioma and benign asbestos pleural effusion. European Journal of Radiology. 2016;**85**:1594–1600.

[14] Paris C, et al. Pleural plaques and asbestosis: Dose- and time-response relationships based on HRCT data. European Respiratory Journal. 2009;**34**:72–79.

[15] Epler GR, et al. Asbestos-related disease from household exposure. Respiration. 1980;**39**:229–240.

[16] Butnor KJ, Sporn TA, Roggli VL. Exposure to brake dust and malignant mesothelioma: A study of 10 cases with mineral fiber analyses. The Annals of Occupational Hygiene. 2003;**47**(4): 325–330.

[17] Nguyen M, et al. CT with histopathologic correlation of FDG uptake in a patient with pulmonary granuloma and pleural plaque caused by remote talc pleurodesis. American Journal of Roentgenology. 2004;**182**: 92–94.

[18] King H. Talc: The Softest Mineral. Geology.com; 2023.

[19] Robinson JJ. Pleural plaques and splenic capsular sclerosis in adult male autopsies. Archives of Pathology. 1972;**93**(2):118–122.

[20] Miller A, et al. Relationship of pulmonary function to radiographic interstitial fibrosis in 2,611 long-term asbestos insulators: An assessment of the International Labour Office profusion score. American Review of Respiratory Disease 1992;**145**:263–270.

[21] Lynch DA, Gamsu G, Aberle DR. Conventional and high resolution computed tomography in the diagnosis of asbestos-related diseases. Radiographics. 1989;**9**(3):523–551.

[22] Huggins JT, Sahn SA. Causes and management of pleural fibrosis. Respirology. 2004;**9**(4):441–447.

[23] Batra P, et al. Rounded atelectasis. Journal of Thoracic Imaging. 1996;**11**:187–197.

[24] Stathopoulos GT, et al. Rounded atelectasis of the lung. Respiratory Medicine. 2005;**99**:615–623.

[25] Ilei P, et al. The use of CDKN2A deletion as a diagnostic marker for malignant mesothelioma in body cavity effusions. Cancer. 2003;**25**:51–56.

[26] Chapel D, et al. MTAP immunohistochemistry is an accurate and reproducible surrogate for CDKN2A fluorescence in situ hybridization in diagnosis of malignant pleural mesothelioma. Moserb Pathology. 2019;**33**:245–254.

[27] Churg A, et al. Malignant mesothelioma in situ. Histopathology. 2018;**72**:1033–1038.

[28] Klebe S, et al. The concept of mesothelioma in situ, with consideration of its potential impact on cytology diagnosis. Pathology. 2021;**53**:446–453.

Chapter 5

Empyema/Fibrothorax

Berivan Karatekin Usta and İlker Kolbaş

Abstract

Pleural infections are a common clinical condition in which hospitalization costs, mortality, and morbidity decrease when treated promptly. The treatment of empyema involves the elimination of the infection source by removing the infected material, facilitating lung expansion, and initiating appropriate antibiotherapy. There is no clear algorithm for the drainage of infected material; the first option may include tube thoracostomy and/or fibrinolytic agents, as well as early thoracoscopic or conventional surgical methods.

Keywords: empyema, fibrothorax, thoracic surgery, VATS, pleural effusion

1. Introduction

Empyema is an ancient clinical problem. Despite the widespread use of antibiotics and vaccination, empyema, which generally occurs due to infectious causes, remains the most prevalent complication of pneumonia and a considerable cause of mortality and morbidity worldwide. The most common causes of empyema are bacterial pneumonia and parapneumonic effusion. Other causes include bronchogenic carcinoma, esophageal rupture, blunt and penetrating thoracic traumas, mediastinitis with pleural extension, bronchogenic or esophageal infected cysts, subdiaphragmatic spread, cervical and thoracic spine infections, and post-surgical etiologies [1].

Nearly 80,000 patients develop empyema each year in the United States and the United Kingdom [2, 3]. The incidence of empyema, which decreased with the initiation of antibiotic use, began to rise again after 1990 [1]. Mortality due to empyema is nearly 20%, and early treatment reduces mortality and morbidity as well as hospital costs [2, 4]. Important factors affecting the development of empyema include alcoholism, malnutrition, immunosuppression (HIV, steroid use, treatment), reflux and aspiration, poor oral hygiene, and chronic lung diseases (COPD, bronchiectasis).

2. Clinical manifestation

The presence of pleural effusion should be investigated in patients with signs and symptoms of pneumonia or with an unexplained manifestation of sepsis, as well as in cases of non-clinical response despite appropriate treatment in community-acquired or hospital-acquired pneumonia [1]. In community-acquired pneumonia,

IntechOpen

complicated parapneumonic effusion and empyema development are associated with alcohol and intravenous drug use, while anaerobic pleural infections are linked to poor oral hygiene and aspiration risk [1]. The development of empyema is a progressive process and is divided into three stages [4].

- Stage 1 (parapneumonic effusion): Exudative fluid **due to increased vascular and pleural permeability** without bacterial organisms, characterized by a low number of WBCs in fluid analysis, a serum liquid LDH ratio of less than 50%, normal pH, and normal glucose levels.

- Stage 2 (fibrinopurulent stage): Fibrin accumulation and loculations occur in the fluid depending on the immune system response. In liquid analysis, pH< 7.20, glucose < 2.2 mmol/L, and LDH >1,000 IU/L. If there is no pus, it is termed complicated parapneumonic effusion and in the presence of pus, it is termed as empyema.

- Stage 3 (chronic organization): This is the subsequent stage; it is characterized by a fibrotic, thick pleural peel that prevents lung expansion by covering the lung, deteriorates lung function, and continues to pose an infection risk. **Bacterial invasion increases the immune response, leading to further neutrophil migration, which kills the microorganisms while increasing CO_2 and lactate levels, thereby initiating a self-perpetuating pathological mechanism** [5].

Staging based on symptoms is not always possible. Clinical manifestations of simple parapneumonic infections and complicated parapneumonic infections are similar. In a randomized controlled study, the median duration of symptoms before admission was reported to be 2 weeks [6]. Pleural effusion should be assessed through chest radiography, computed tomography (CT), and pleural ultrasonography (USG). The minimum amount of fluid that can be detected in conventional posteroanterior (PA) chest radiography is 200 mL; however, occasionally, fluids up to 500 mL may not be observed on direct radiography (**Figure 1**) [7].

CT examination serves as a valuable tool in detecting parenchymal, bronchial, and esophageal pathologies, as well as assessing the pleural space. It also aids in differentiating pleural-based lung abscesses from empyema [8]. CT can be utilized not only for diagnosis but also for monitoring cases where clinical improvement is delayed or requires further evaluation [9]. Typically, lenticular-shaped fluid collections, formed by compression of the adjacent lung parenchyma, suggest localized empyema and can be distinguished from pleural-based lung abscesses [1]. Pleural free fluid may not be observed in empyema due to adhesions between the visceral and parietal pleura [7]. Pleural thickening and enhancement are seen in the vast majority of patients with empyema; simultaneous thickening and enhancement of both the visceral and parietal pleura strongly indicate empyema. In addition, a decrease in intrapleural fatty tissue and the presence of a split pleura sign are observed [1]. Moreover, spontaneous air bubbles within pleural effusion are associated with pleural fluid infection [10].

Positron emission tomography (PET/CT) and magnetic resonance imaging (MRI) can be useful in determining fluid characteristics (**Figure 2**) [11, 12].

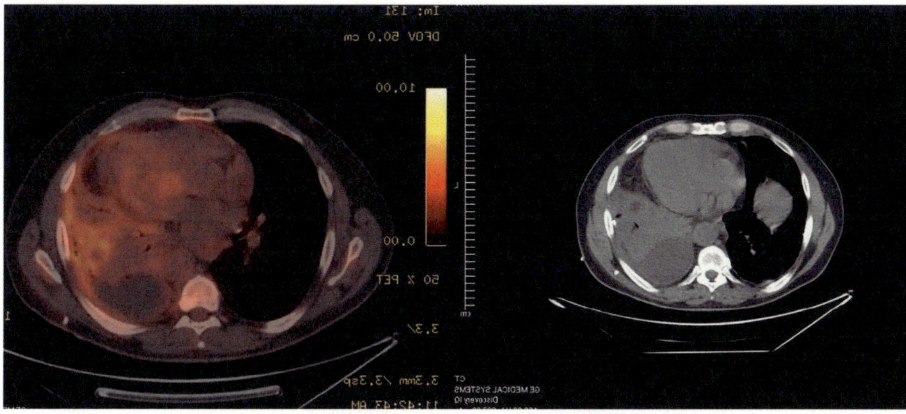

Figure 1.
PET/CT scan of patient with empyema.

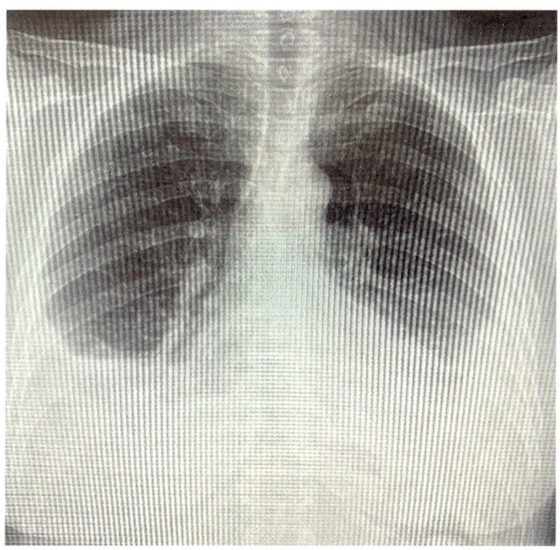

Figure 2.
Patient with bilateral pleural effusion.

Pleural USG has been widely used in recent years thanks to its advantages, such as rapid evaluation of the patient in emergency and intensive care units, its ability to be applied at the bedside, its greater sensitivity compared to conventional radiographs in the evaluation of pleural fluids, the fact that it does not require a radiologist, and its capability to determine whether the fluid is complicated and contains septa based on the echogenicity of the fluid (**Figure 3**) [13, 14].

3. Thoracentesis

Diagnostic pleural sampling is imperative in pleural effusions associated with sepsis or pneumonia because pleural effusion detected in radiological examination

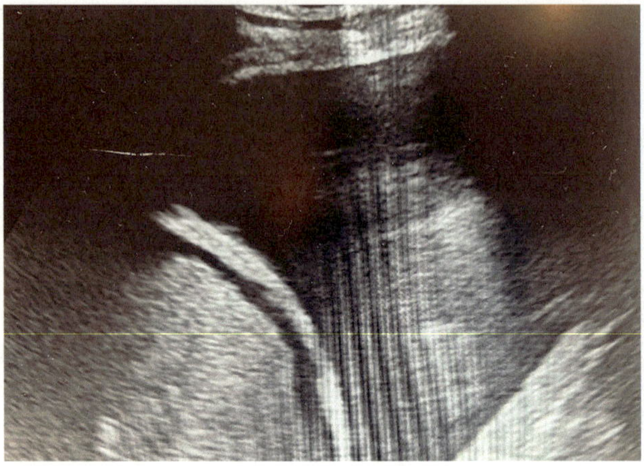

Figure 3.
USG image of pleural effusion.

can evolve into pleural infection, and detection of it is clinically impossible [2]. To reduce the risk of pneumothorax in thoracentesis, the indication for thoracentesis is identified in suspected pleural effusions with fluid presence of 2.5 cm or more in a 1 cm thorax CT on direct radiography [1, 15]. At least 25–50 mL of pleural fluid should be taken for cytological examination during thoracentesis. If infection is suspected, collecting samples in blood culture bottles increases culture efficiency [9].

Ultrasonography-guided puncture should be performed [16]. The risk of iatrogenic pneumothorax following thoracentesis ranges between 0.61% and 6.0%. Symptoms of pneumothorax that develop after the procedure usually occur 1–4 hours later, so the patient should be followed up, and if symptoms develop, chest radiography should be performed and examined [17].

A multidisciplinary approach (chest medicine, thoracic surgery, infectious diseases, radiology) is important in patient management. This multidisciplinary approach enhances patient safety in diagnostic procedures, surgical decision-making, and follow-up decisions. In acute empyema, antibiotherapy is determined by considering the patient's clinical history, local and institutional antibiotherapy management protocols, and culture results. Second- or third-generation cephalosporins or aminopenicillin/ß-lactamase inhibitor combinations, which are administered as first-line treatments in community-acquired pneumonia and empyema, are effective treatments for strains that are common in the community [18]. Anaerobic organisms should be treated empirically. Although aerobic growth may occur in cultures, anaerobic agents should be added to the medication regimen due to the possibility of anaerobic culture failure and the likelihood of empyema being infected with anaerobic microorganisms [18]. Although ampicillin/sulbactam is effective against various anaerobes, it requires the addition of an agent such as metronidazole when using ceftriaxone. Clindamycin is an appropriate alternative to metronidazole, as it is effective against many anaerobic agents [19].

In hospital-acquired or surgery-related infections, the combination of cefepime–vancomycin and Flagyl, or vancomycin and piperacillin/tazobactam, which will also

(a) (b)

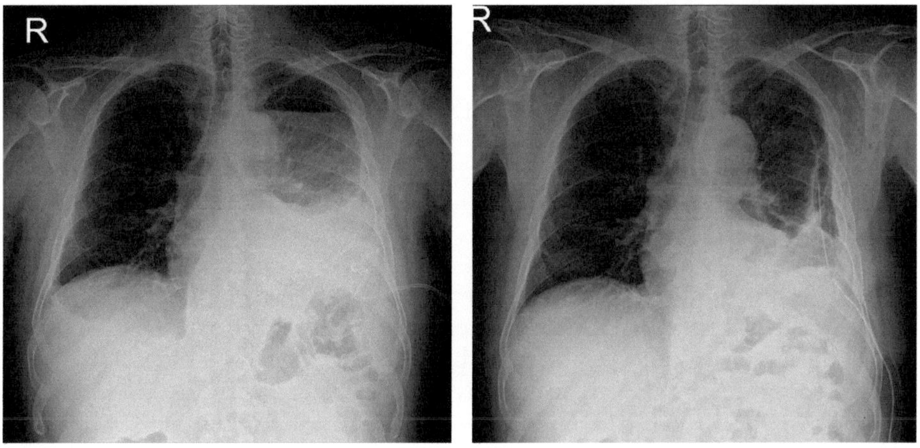

Figure 4.
(a) 14 F catheter and (b) chest tube.

be effective against methicillin-resistant *Staphylococcus aureus* and *Pseudomonas*, should be preferred until the culture results are obtained [1]. Treatment for empyema lasts 2–6 weeks after drainage and abatement of fever. The duration of treatment varies depending on the drug resistance status of the microorganism causing the infection, the efficiency of the drainage, and the containment of the infection source.

Drainage of infected material is the mainstay of empyema treatment. Although cases of empyema treated with therapeutic thoracentesis and antibiotherapy have been reported, to date, no randomized controlled studies demonstrating the superiority of repeated thoracentesis, tube thoracostomy, or early VATS procedures have been conducted [3]. Tube thoracostomy and antibiotherapy should be performed in the treatment of early-stage empyema [4]. There is no consensus on the preferred catheter diameters for pleural drainage (**Figure 4A-4B**). In small-diameter catheters, drain blockage is more common than in large-diameter catheters, but the blockage can be overcome by flushing with saline solution. If drainage cannot be ensured with small-caliber drains, placing a second drain or a larger-caliber drain may ensure drainage [4, 20–23].

4. Fibrinolytic therapy

Intrapleural fibrinolytics are used for the separation of fibrous septations and drainage of fibrinopurulent empyema in empyema and complicated parapneumonic effusion [1]. It has been demonstrated that intrapleural streptokinase increases the amount of pleural fluid drainage but has no effect on fibrinolysis, mortality, operation frequency, or duration of hospital stay [6, 24]. The use of a combination of intrapleural tissue plasminogen activator (t-PA) and DNase has been shown to reduce pleural drainage, duration of hospital stay, and the need for surgery [25].

Studies comparing the use of tube thoracostomy and fibrinolytic agents with the use of VATS as the first treatment in the management of fibrinopurulent empyema have shown higher success rates, shorter tube duration, and reduced hospitalization duration in the VATS group [26–28]. However, fibrinolytic therapy appears to be the most ideal choice for patients with contraindications to surgery.

5. Surgery

Surgery is recommended in cases where tube thoracostomy is inefficient, the presence of pleural fluid cannot be drained, and empyema progresses and causes fibrosis [3]. Surgery should be preferred in the third stage of empyema since pleural drainage procedures would not be effective [1]. It has been revealed in the literature that surgery is the best approach to choose as the first-line treatment for empyema [29, 30]. The primary goals of surgical intervention are debridement of the pleural space and lung expansion [1, 3, 4]. All loculations in the pleural space should be opened, all fluid should be drained, and pleural thickening and infected tissue that cause the lung to collapse should be decorticated to ensure expansion. If the parenchyma does not cause sepsis or has hemoptysis, the necrotic parenchyma should be resected [31].

Surgical treatment of empyema can be categorized as decortication, decortication with lobectomy and/or pneumonectomy, closure of the pleural cavities, and open drainage of the empyema space. If necessary, more than one procedure can be applied to the same patient [31].

The concept of decortication involves the resection of the organized visceral and parietal pleura by stripping, thereby enabling the re-expansion of the lung. The success of the procedure is related to the extent of damage to the parenchyma throughout the operation [31]. Surgery can be performed using video-assisted thoracoscopic surgery (VATS) or conventional thoracotomy. In cases of empyema with loculated contours, the location of the thoracotomy incision can be determined preoperatively, making access to the empyema sac easier. Extrapleural decortication during thoracotomy is a rapid, time-saving procedure [3]. The literature has shown that VATS is superior to thoracotomy in terms of postoperative pain, blood loss, duration of hospitalization, and cost in the treatment of pulmonary, pleural, esophageal, and mediastinal diseases [32–34]. It has been suggested that thoracoscopic decortication can be performed with lower mortality and morbidity rates [35, 36]. The success of VATS has been reported to correlate with surgical experience and expertise [37]. The need to convert from VATS to thoracotomy is associated with factors such as the stage of the disease, the duration of symptom onset, male gender, postpneumonic empyema, and the presence of gram-negative microorganisms [38, 39]. Operation duration has been identified as the most significant independent risk factor affecting the likelihood of conversion to thoracotomy [39–41]. However, VATS has been demonstrated to be as effective as open decortication in the treatment of Stage 3 disease [37, 38].

Omentum or muscle flaps can be used to prevent the accumulation of infected fluid in the absence of full expansion during the operation or the resection of the necrotic lung parenchyma [42, 43]. While thoracotomy is

DOI: http://dx.doi.org/10.5772/intechopen.1012706

needed for muscle flaps, the thoracoscopy technique can be used for an omentum flap [42]. Any extrathoracic muscle can be preferred for muscle flaps; the most commonly used muscles are the serratus anterior, latissimus dorsi, and pectoralis major [43].

Other ways to reduce the thoracic cavity include pleural tent and thoracoplasty [31, 44]. Decortication, with or without parenchymal resection, in patients with chronic empyema may result in a large infected area that needs to be controlled in the presence of bronchopleural fistula (BPF). Creating an open thoracic window with rib resection allows the infected cavity to be debrided and facilitates the formation of granulation tissue. In recent years, studies have shown better tissue debridement and granulation groove formation through vacuum-assisted closure (VAC) of the infected cavity [45]. Care should be taken when using VAC in the presence of BPF or a significant air leak in the visceral pleura.

The rate of empyema developing after surgery is 2%–16%. Empyema associated with BPF is generally identified after pneumonectomy, and there are a small number of reported cases of empyema after lobectomy. Risk factors for BPF include having benign disease, right pneumonectomy, completion pneumonectomy, a diagnosis of diabetes mellitus (DM), tuberculosis, resection following neoadjuvant chemoradiotherapy, and enlarged lymph node dissection [46, 47]. Empyema cases developing after pneumonectomy are generally accompanied by BPF, and mortality rates have been reported as 28%–50% in the literature [48]. In empyema cases developing after pneumonectomy, the presence of BPF should be investigated as a priority, and fiberoptic bronchoscopy (FOB) should be performed to verify the presence of BPF. Until the presence of a fistula is excluded, tube thoracostomy should be applied as a first-line treatment to contain the infection and prevent contralateral spread, assuming that BPF is present in all cases. For drainage of the pleural space, the patient is placed in a lateral decubitus position with the pneumonectomy side down, and appropriate antibiotherapy is initiated [1].

There are few studies in which bronchoscopic interventions for fistula closure in the presence of BPF have been successful [49, 50]. More invasive techniques, such as the Clagett procedure, modified Clagett procedure, or open-window thoracostomy, may be required in resistant cases. The Clagett procedure involves the drainage of the infected pleural cavity, bathing it with an antibiotic solution, cleaning the infection, then filling the whole hemithorax with the antibiotic solution, and finally closing the thorax with a second operation [51]. As treatment failure is typically caused by ongoing or recurrent fistula, the pneumonectomy stump has been modified to prevent ischemia and necrosis by supporting it with a well-vascularized flap, and empyema can be successfully treated [52–54].

In the treatment of patients with empyema secondary to resection, opening a thoracostomy window, filling the cavity with antibiotic solution after the infection has been effectively treated, and obliteration of the residual space with muscle or omentum may be preferred [51–54].

Author details

Berivan Karatekin Usta[1] and İlker Kolbaş[2]*

1 Department of Chest Diseases, Istanbul Aydın University, Istanbul, Türkiye

2 Department of Thoracic Surgery, Istanbul Aydın University, Istanbul, Türkiye

*Address all correspondence to: dr_ilkerkolbas@hotmail.com

References

[1] Shen KR, Bribriesco A, Crabtree T, et al. The American Association for Thoracic surgery consensus guidelines for the management of empyema. The Journal of Thoracic and Cardiovascular Surgery. 2017;**153**(6):e129–e146. DOI: 10.1016/j.jtcvs.2017.01.030

[2] Finley C, Clifton J, Fitzgerald JM, Yee J. Empyema: An increasing concern in Canada. Canadian Respiratory Journal. 2008;**15**(2):85–89. DOI: 10.1155/2008/975312

[3] Scarci M, Abah U, Solli P, et al. EACTS expert consensus statement for surgical management of pleural empyema. European Journal of Cardio-Thoracic Surgery. 2015;**48**(5):642–653. DOI: 10.1093/ejcts/ezv272

[4] Davies HE, Davies RJO, Davies CWH, on behalf of the BTS Pleural Disease Guideline Group. Management of pleural infection in adults: British Thoracic Society pleural disease guideline 2010. Thorax. 2010;**65**(Suppl 2):ii41–ii53. DOI: 10.1136/thx.2010.137000

[5] Maskell NA, Davies CWH, Nunn AJ, et al. U.K. Controlled Trial of Intrapleural Streptokinase for Pleural Infection. New England Journal of Medicine. 2005;**352**(9):865–874. DOI: 10.1056/NEJMoa042473

[6] Hallifax RJ, Talwar A, Wrightson JM, Edey A, Gleeson FV. State-of-the-art: Radiological investigation of pleural disease. Respiratory Medicine. 2017;**124**:88–99. DOI: 10.1016/j.rmed.2017.02.013

[7] Stark D, Federle M, Goodman P, Podrasky A, Webb W. Differentiating lung abscess and empyema: Radiography and computed tomography. American Journal of Roentgenology. 1983;**141**(1):163–167. DOI: 10.2214/ajr.141.1.163

[8] Smolikov A, Smolyakov R, Riesenberg K, et al. Prevalence and clinical significance of pleural microbubbles in computed tomography of thoracic empyema. Clinical Radiology. 2006;**61**(6):513–519. DOI: 10.1016/j.crad.2006.02.004

[9] Yang M-F, Tong Z-H, Wang Z, et al. Development and validation of the PET-CT score for diagnosis of malignant pleural effusion. European Journal of Nuclear Medicine and Molecular Imaging. 2019;**46**(7):1457–1467. DOI: 10.1007/s00259-019-04287-7

[10] Liszewski MC, Ciet P, Lee EY. Lung and Pleura. Pediatric Body MRI. Published online May 24, **2020**:1–28

[11] Asciak R, Hassan M, Mercer RM, et al. Prospective analysis of the predictive value of sonographic pleural fluid Echogenicity for the diagnosis of exudative effusion. Respiration. 2019;**97**(5):451–456. DOI: 10.1159/000496153

[12] Yang PC, Luh KT, Chang DB, Wu HD, Yu CJ, Kuo SH. Value of sonography in determining the nature of pleural effusion: Analysis of 320 cases. American Journal of Roentgenology. 1992;**159**(1):29–33. DOI: 10.2214/ajr.159.1.1609716

[13] Moffett BK, Panchabhai TS, Anaya E, et al. Computed tomography measurements of parapneumonic effusion indicative of thoracentesis. European Respiratory Journal. 2011;**38**

(6):1406–1411. DOI: 10.1183/09031936.00004511

[14] Havelock T, Teoh R, Laws D, Gleeson F, BTS Pleural Disease Guideline Group. Pleural procedures and thoracic ultrasound: British Thoracic society pleural disease guideline 2010. Thorax. 2010;**65** (Suppl 2):ii61–76. DOI: 10.1136/thx.2010.137026

[15] Jany B, Welte T. Pleural effusion in adults—etiology, diagnosis, and treatment. Deutsches Arzteblatt International. 2019;**116**(21):377–386. DOI: 10.3238/arztebl.2019.0377

[16] Metlay JP, Waterer GW, Long AC, et al. Diagnosis and treatment of adults with community-acquired Pneumonia. An official clinical practice guideline of the American thoracic society and infectious diseases society of America. American Journal of Respiratory and Critical Care Medicine. 2019;**200**(7): e45–e67. DOI: 10.1164/rccm.201908-1581ST

[17] Brook I, Wexler HM, Goldstein EJC. Antianaerobic antimicrobials: Spectrum and susceptibility testing. Clinical Microbiology Reviews. 2013;**26** (3):526–546. DOI: 10.1128/CMR.00086-12

[18] Rahman NM, Maskell NA, Davies CWH, et al. The relationship between chest tube size and clinical outcome in pleural infection. Chest. 2010;**137** (3):536–543. DOI: 10.1378/chest.09-1044

[19] Davies HE, Merchant S, McGown A. A study of the complications of small bore "Seldinger" intercostal chest drains. Respirology. 2008;**13**(4): 603–607. DOI: 10.1111/j.1440-1843.2008.01296.x

[20] Cafarotti S, Dall'Armi V, Cusumano G, et al. Small-bore wire-guided chest drains: Safety, tolerability, and effectiveness in pneumothorax, malignant effusions, and pleural empyema. The Journal of Thoracic and Cardiovascular Surgery. 2011;**141** (3):683–687. DOI: 10.1016/j.jtcvs.2010.08.044

[21] Yu H. Management of pleural effusion, Empyema, and lung abscess. Seminars in Interventional Radiology. 2011;**28**(1):75–86. DOI: 10.1055/s-0031-1273942

[22] Tokuda Y, Matsushima D, Stein GH, Miyagi S. Intrapleural fibrinolytic agents for empyema and complicated parapneumonic effusions: A meta-analysis. Chest. 2006;**129**(3):783–790. DOI: 10.1378/chest.129.3.783

[23] Rahman NM, Phil D, Maskell NA, et al. Intrapleural use of tissue plasminogen activator and DNAse in pleural infection. The New England Journal of Medicine. 2011;**365**(6):518–26

[24] Wait MA, Sharma S, Hohn J, Dal Nogare A. A randomized trial of empyema therapy. Chest. 1997;**111** (6):1548–1551. DOI: 10.1378/chest.111.6.1548

[25] Petrakis IE, Kogerakis NE, Drositis IE, Lasithiotakis KG, Bouros D, Chalkiadakis GE. Video-assisted thoracoscopic surgery for thoracic Empyema: Primarily, or after fibrinolytic therapy failure? The American Journal of Surgery. 2004;**187** (4):471–474. DOI: 10.1016/j.amjsurg.2003.12.048

[26] Muhammad MIA. Management of complicated parapneumonic effusion and empyema using different treatment modalities. Asian Cardiovascular and

Thoracic Annals. 2012;**20**(2):177–181. DOI: 10.1177/0218492311435338

[27] Shin JA, Chang YS, Kim TH, et al. Surgical decortication as the first-line treatment for pleural empyema. The Journal of Thoracic and Cardiovascular Surgery. 2013;**145**(4):933–939.e1. DOI: 10.1016/j.jtcvs.2012.07.035

[28] Chen K-C, Chen H-Y, Lin J-W, et al. Acute thoracic empyema: Clinical characteristics and outcome analysis of video-assisted thoracoscopic surgery. Journal of the Formosan Medical Association. 2014;**113**(4):210–218. DOI: 10.1016/j.jfma.2013.12.010

[29] Shiraishi Y. Surgical treatment of chronic empyema. General Thoracic and Cardiovascular Surgery. 2010;**58** (7):311–316. DOI: 10.1007/s11748-010-0599-6

[30] Chambers A, Routledge T, Dunning J, Scarci M. Is video-assisted thoracoscopic surgical decortication superior to open surgery in the management of adults with primary empyema? Interactive CardioVascular and Thoracic Surgery. 2010;**11**(2): 171–177. DOI: 10.1510/icvts.2010.240408

[31] Farjah F, Backhus LM, Varghese TK, et al. Ninety-day costs of video-assisted thoracic surgery versus open lobectomy for lung cancer. The Annals of Thoracic Surgery. 2014;**98**(1): 191–196. DOI: 10.1016/j.athoracsur.2014.03.024

[32] Watson TJ, Qiu J. The impact of Thoracoscopic surgery on payment and health care utilization after lung resection. The Annals of Thoracic Surgery. 2016;**101**(4):1271–1279. discussion 1979-1980. DOI:10.1016/j.athoracsur.2015.10.104

[33] Tsai C-H, Lai Y-C, Chang S-C, Chang C-Y, Wang W-S, Yuan M-K. Video-assisted thoracoscopic surgical decortication in the elderly with thoracic empyema: Five years' experience. Journal of the Chinese Medical Association. 2016;**79**(1): 25–28. DOI: 10.1016/j.jcma.2015.06.013

[34] Bongiolatti S, Voltolini L, Borgianni S, et al. Uniportal thoracoscopic decortication for pleural empyema and the role of ultrasonographic preoperative staging†. Interactive CardioVascular and Thoracic Surgery. 2017:ivw423. DOI: 10.1093/icvts/ivw423

[35] Shahin Y, Duffy J, Beggs D, Black E, Majewski A. Surgical management of primary empyema of the pleural cavity: Outcome of 81 patients. Interactive CardioVascular and Thoracic Surgery. 2010;**10**(4):565–567. DOI: 10.1510/icvts.2009.215004

[36] Chung JH, Lee SH, Kim KT, Jung JS, Son HS, Sun K. Optimal timing of thoracoscopic drainage and decortication for empyema. The Annals of Thoracic Surgery. 2014;**97**(1): 224–229. DOI: 10.1016/j.athoracsur.2013.08.039

[37] Lardinois D, Gock M, Pezzetta E, et al. Delayed referral and gram-negative organisms increase the conversion thoracotomy rate in patients undergoing video-assisted thoracoscopic surgery for empyema. The Annals of Thoracic Surgery. 2005;**79**(6):1851–1856. DOI: 10.1016/j.athoracsur.2004.12.031

[38] Da W, R A.Thoracoscopic decortication: A role for video-assisted surgery in chronic postpneumonic pleural empyema. The Annals of

Thoracic Surgery. 2001;**71**(6). DOI: 10.1016/s0003-4975(01)02471-7

[39] Stefani A, Aramini B, Della Casa G, et al. Preoperative predictors of successful surgical treatment in the management of parapneumonic empyema. The Annals of Thoracic Surgery. 2013;**96**(5):1812–1819. DOI: 10.1016/j.athoracsur.2013.06.013

[40] Endoh H, Yamamoto R, Nishizawa N, Satoh Y. Thoracoscopic surgery using omental flap for bronchopleural fistula. Surgical Case Reports. 2019;**5**(1):5. DOI: 10.1186/s40792-019-0563-3

[41] Shinohara S, Chikaishi Y, Kuwata T, et al. Benefits of using omental pedicle flap over muscle flap for closure of open window thoracotomy. Journal of Thoracic Disease. 2016;**8**(7):1697–1703. DOI: 10.21037/jtd.2016.05.91

[42] Botianu PV-H, Botianu AM. Thoracomyoplasty in the Treatment of Empyema: Current Indications, Basic Principles, and Results. Pulmonary Medicine. 2012;**2012**:1–6. DOI: 10.1155/2012/418514

[43] Hofmann H-S, Schemm R, Grosser C, Szöke T, Sziklavari Z. Vacuum-assisted closure of pleural empyema without classic open-window thoracostomy. The Annals of Thoracic Surgery. 2012;**93**(5):1741–1742. DOI: 10.1016/j.athoracsur.2011.12.039

[44] Deschamps C, Bernard A, Nichols FC, et al. Empyema and bronchopleural fistula after pneumonectomy: Factors affecting incidence. The Annals of Thoracic Surgery. 2001;**72**(1):243–247. discussion 248. DOI: 10.1016/s0003-4975(01)02681-9

[45] Llewellyn-Bennett R, Wotton R, West D. Prophylactic flap coverage and the incidence of bronchopleural fistulae after pneumonectomy. Interactive CardioVascular and Thoracic Surgery. 2013;**16**(5):681–685. DOI: 10.1093/icvts/ivt002

[46] Sivrikoz MC, Elbeyli L Cerrahi Sonras› Ampiyemler. Published online 2002:6

[47] Klotz LV, Gesierich W, Schott-Hildebrand S, Hatz RA, Lindner M. Endobronchial closure of bronchopleural fistula using Amplatzer device. Journal of Thoracic Disease. 2015;**7**(8):1478–1482. DOI: 10.3978/j.issn.2072-1439.2015.08.25

[48] Marwah V, Katoch CDS, Kumar K, Pathak K, Bhattacharjee S, Jindamwar P. Bronchoscopic device closure of postoperative bronchopleural fistulae: Novel devices and innovative techniques. Lung India: Official Organ of Indian Chest Society. 2020;**37**(2):107–113. DOI: 10.4103/lungindia.lungindia_179_19

[49] Borges N, Saha S. Thoracoplasty for postpneumonectomy Empyema Associated with Bronchopleural Fistula: A case series. The International Journal of Angiology : Official Publication of the International College of Angiology, Inc. 2015;**24**(2):151–154. DOI: 10.1055/s-0034-1370886

[50] Pairolero PC, Arnold PG, Trastek VF, Meland NB, Kay PP, Postpneumonectomy empyema. The role of intrathoracic muscle transposition. The Journal of Thoracic and Cardiovascular Surgery. 1990;**99**(6):958–966. discussion 966-968

[51] Wojcik J, Grodzki T, Kubisa B, Pierog J, Safranow K, Naprawa G. Accelerated treatment of postpneumonectomy empyema - report

of 12-year experience. Neoplasma. 2013;**60**(2):160–166. DOI: 10.4149/neo_2013_021

[52] Zaheer S, Allen MS, Cassivi SD, et al. Postpneumonectomy empyema: Results after the Clagett procedure. The Annals of Thoracic Surgery. 2006;**82**(1):279–286. discussion 286-287. DOI: 10.1016/j.athoracsur.2006.01.052

[53] S D, G T, L D, et al. Accelerated treatment of postpneumonectomy empyema: A binational long-term study. The Journal of Thoracic and Cardiovascular Surgery. 2008;**136**(1):179–185. DOI: 10.1016/j.jtcvs.2008.01.036

[54] Eloesser L. Of an operation for Tuberculous Empyema. The Annals of Thoracic Surgery. 1969;**8**(4):355–357. DOI: 10.1016/S0003-4975(10)66250-9

Section 3

Diagnostic Advances in Pleural Disease

Chapter 6

Lung Cancer Driver Mutation Testing Using Pleural Effusion

Hsin-Yi Wang and Jin-Yuan Shih

Abstract

Pleural effusion fluid has been established as a highly informative substrate for non-small cell lung cancer (NSCLC) genotyping. Current evidence demonstrates that mutations in *EGFR*, *ALK*, *ROS1*, *BRAF*, *KRAS*, *MET*, *RET*, *HER2*, *NTRK*, and other clinically relevant genes can be accurately identified by analyzing DNA from pleural fluid supernatants, small cytology specimens, or cell blocks. Pleural fluid molecular testing demonstrates high sensitivity, comparable to tissue biopsy, and consistently outperforms traditional plasma-based liquid biopsies. Specificity is also excellent, with mutations identified in pleural fluid strongly correlating with treatment responses and patient outcomes, underscoring their clinical validity. Pleural effusion cell blocks are valuable for both histological diagnosis and genotyping, providing a less invasive and reliable method to detect major actionable mutations, with diagnostic performance approaching that of conventional tissue biopsies. Successful molecular analysis using cell blocks depends on adequate tumor cell content and sensitive detection techniques to maximize mutation identification. Moreover, cell-free DNA (cfDNA) obtained from pleural fluid supernatants has emerged as an especially rich source of tumor DNA, even in cytology-negative or paucicellular samples. Next-generation sequencing (NGS) of pleural cfDNA achieves diagnostic yields comparable to tissue biopsies and superior to pleural cytology and plasma cfDNA. Current clinical guidelines recommend the use of cytology specimens or liquid biopsies for molecular testing in lung cancer, reflecting a paradigm shift toward utilizing all available sample types to guide therapeutic decisions. Thus, pleural effusion represents an ideal alternative substrate for NSCLC genomic testing, particularly when tissue biopsy is not feasible.

Keywords: pleural effusion, NSCLC, cfDNA, ctDNA, next-generation sequencing, liquid biopsy

1. Introduction

At the time of diagnosis, 15% of lung cancer patients have pleural effusions, and over time, this rate may increase to 50% [1]. Adenocarcinoma is the most common lung cancer type, causing malignant pleural effusion. Malignant pleural effusion (MPE) is defined by the detection of malignant cells in the pleural fluid. The presence of MPE denotes systemic dissemination of cancer and meets the criteria for M1a disease, as per the American Joint Committee on Cancer TNM. On the other hand, paramalignant effusions are pleural effusions found in patients with solid tumors without direct pleural involvement and no evidence of malignant cells in the pleural fluid [2]. Common causes responsible for the development of paramalignant effusion include lymphatic obstruction, pulmonary embolism, bronchial obstruction, and complications of radiation and chemotherapy.

The treatment setting for non–small cell lung cancer (NSCLC) has been transformed by the impressive clinical activity of targeted therapies. Over the past decade, an expanding list of genomic alterations in NSCLC has become "druggable" with targeted therapies. The College of American Pathologists (CAP), the International Association for the Study of Lung Cancer (IASLC), and the Association for Molecular Pathology (AMP) molecular testing guideline strongly recommend testing all advanced NSCLC adenocarcinoma patients for at least *EGFR*, *ALK*, and *ROS1*, and suggest including *BRAF*, *MET*, *RET*, *HER2*, and *KRAS* as part of larger panels, especially if initial tests are negative [3]. The National Comprehensive Cancer Network treatment guidelines also recommend broad molecular testing for patients with lung cancer to identify those who would benefit from available or emerging targeted therapies in clinical trials [4]. Molecular testing in lung adenocarcinoma has traditionally relied on tissue specimens from biopsy or surgical resection. However, obtaining adequate tissue biopsy specimens for NSCLC is becoming increasingly challenging owing to the growing number of biomarkers; inadequate tumor samples for comprehensive molecular analysis are common [5, 6]. There is an urgent need to identify other biological materials from patients that can substitute for tumor tissues, since tumor tissue samples are not always available.

Although invasive tissue biopsy remains the diagnostic gold standard due to its high sensitivity and specificity, non-invasive biomarker analysis using pleural effusion is rapidly closing the gap. In this article, we summarize the clinical utility of pleural effusion for detecting driver mutations in NSCLC.

2. Analytical approaches for pleural effusion analysis

Pleural effusion fluid contains valuable tumor-derived materials. Once drained, the fluid sample is typically centrifuged and separated into a cellular fraction (cell pellet) and a cell-free supernatant. Various laboratory techniques can be used to detect driver mutations, including cytological examination, DNA – and RNA-based assays (such as Sanger sequencing, amplification refractory mutation system (ARMS-PCR), mutant-specific polymerase chain reaction (PCR), digital PCR, and next-generation sequencing (NGS)), liquid biopsy methods for cell-free DNA (cfDNA), and even exploratory proteomic or cellular analyses. An efficient workflow involves dividing the pleural fluid into parallel processes, with the cell pellet utilized for cytology, potentially immunocytochemistry (IHC) and molecular testing, and the supernatant allocated for molecular testing [7] (**Figure 1**).

Improvements in the analytical sensitivity of sequencing platforms, such as digital PCR and NGS, have enabled the detection of mutant alleles at very low levels. This progress has facilitated genomic analysis from smaller, even paucicellular samples, expanding the options for molecular testing [8–10]. Consequently, cytology samples have become increasingly valuable for genomic

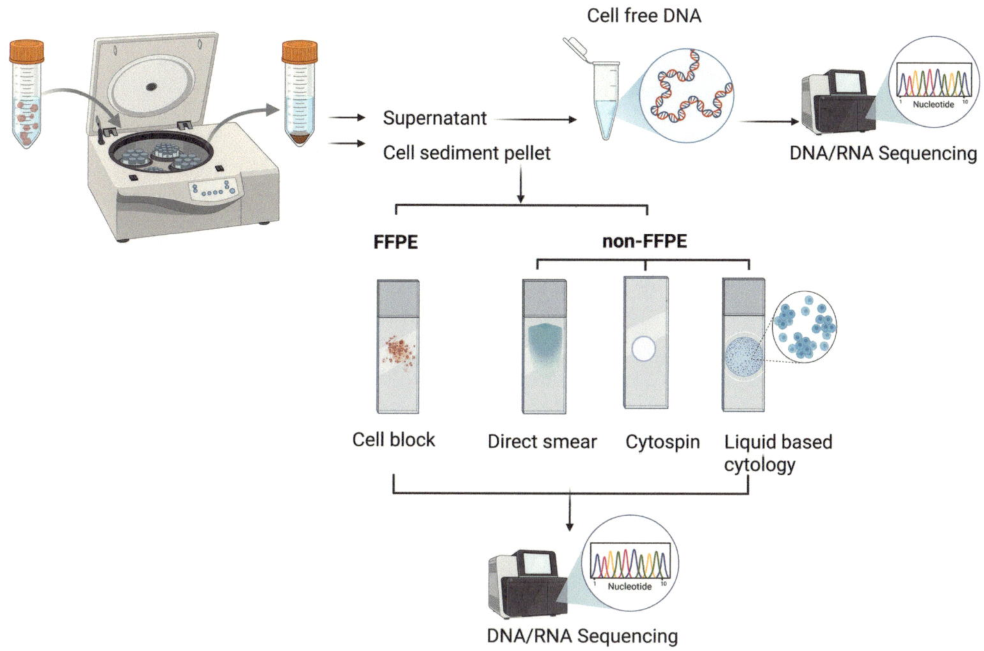

Figure 1.
Analytical approaches for pleural effusion in driver mutation detection in NSCLC.

analysis due to their accessibility, safety, and cost-effectiveness associated with minimally invasive sampling methods [11]. Additionally, liquid biopsy using cfDNA has also been extensively studied and is a widely adopted alternative to tissue tumor genotyping. Pleural fluid has emerged as an alternative "liquid biopsy" source of tumor DNA and cells. It has been found that pleural fluid samples are often highly informative for tumor genetics. In fact, pleural fluid can sometimes yield more tumor DNA than small tissue biopsies [12]. Because pleural fluids are readily accessible through minimally invasive techniques, direct use of effusion samples for genomic analysis reduces the need for more invasive procedures and expands the opportunity for molecular diagnosis to more patients. Pleural effusions have proven to be invaluable sources for detecting driver mutations in NSCLC, especially when conventional tissue samples are limited or unavailable [13]. Descriptions of various pleural effusion sample types are provided in the following section, and a comparison of these samples is presented in **Table 1**.

3. Non–formalin-fixed, paraffin-embedded cytology

Pleural fluid cells are commonly processed into cell blocks for IHC and DNA extraction. However, alternative cytology preparations – including direct smears, liquid-based cytology (LBC) slides, and cytospin preparations – are increasingly utilized for molecular testing. Regular use of cytology samples in molecular testing remains challenging due to a paucity of tumor cells and a high degree of cellular

Specimens	Tumor		Pleural effusion	
	Tissue	**Cell sediment cytology**	**Cell block**	**CfDNA**
Invasiveness	Invasive	Less invasive	Less invasive	Less invasive
Tumor DNA amount	Abundant if adequate specimens	Requires malignant cells; often low due to limited cellularity	Requires malignant cells; moderate to high	Tumor DNA present even without malignant cells
Diagnostic yield	High; Gold standard	Moderate; variable depends on cellularity	Moderately high; approaches tissue biopsy if adequate cellularity	High; comparable to tissue biopsy. Outperforms plasma cfDNA
Advantage	1. Gold standard 2. Histology information	1. Faster turnaround and flexibility 2. No formalin-related nucleic acid damage	1. Repeat sampling was possible to track clonal evolution 2. Histology information	1. Repeat sampling was possible to track clonal evolution 2. Capture tumor heterogeneity
Limitation	1. Longer turnaround time 2. Tissue biopsy is not always feasible	1. Low cellularity 2. Inadequate for comprehensive genomic profiling	1. Occasional low cellularity	1. High-level technical requirements 2. Lack of histology information
Clinical utility	Standard of care; Well standardized	Adjunctive; Less standardized	Widely adopted in routine diagnostics; well standardized	Increasingly adopted in specialized centers; ongoing development for standardization and generalization

Table 1.
Comparison of tissue biopsy, pleural effusion cytology, cell block, and pleural effusion cfDNA in NSCLC driver mutation detection.

heterogeneity [14]. Malignant effusions, however, often provide abundant tumor cells, generating sufficient cell pellets suitable for DNA/RNA extraction or smear preparation. Multiple studies have confirmed the feasibility of detecting mutations using pleural effusion cell sediment pellets [15, 16]. Guidelines from the CAP/IASLC/AMP explicitly state that cytology specimens are acceptable for molecular testing and should be used when tissue is limited [17].

There are several practical and clinical advantages to utilizing direct cytology preparations from pleural effusions, including the avoidance of invasive procedures, faster turnaround, and greater flexibility. Another advantage of direct cytology samples is that they are not formalin-fixed and often undergo faster and gentler fixation using ethanol-based methods or air-drying, resulting in less fragmented nucleic acids compared to formalin-fixed paraffin-embedded (FFPE) tissue [18]. Formalin fixation leads to chemical cross-links with proteins, RNA, and other DNA molecules, along with concomitant fragmentation of DNA, which inhibits molecular analysis in a length-dependent fashion [17]. Formalin fixation also causes random nucleotide base changes, which can lead to false-positive results, particularly in samples with low DNA concentration or when using ultrasensitive assays [17, 19]. Direct cytology preparations may confer better quality nucleic acids for molecular assays. Additionally, higher-quality RNA can be obtained from fresh pleural fluid cells, facilitating fusion detection, whereas FFPE cell blocks often yield fragmented RNA [20, 21].

There remained some limitations and challenges associated with using non-cell block cytology samples for molecular testing. The accuracy of mutation detection is directly tied to having enough tumor cells and DNA in the sample. Some pleural effusions, especially after therapy, may have very few malignant cells amidst abundant inflammatory cells. A negative result in such a scenario could be a false-negative due to scant tumor DNA.

Unlike FFPE blocks, which follow relatively standardized processing, cytology samples have variable preparation methods and unique pre-analytical variables, such as different fixatives, stains, and storage conditions, that must be managed to ensure reliable results [22]. Cytology specimens processed with heavy metal fixatives (e.g., Zenker, B5, B plus, acid zinc formalin) or acidic solutions (e.g., Bouin solution, bone-decalcifying solutions) should be avoided in DNA-based molecular assays, as heavy metals interfere with enzymatic reactions used in molecular methods, and acidic solutions cause extensive DNA degradation [17]. Most cytology fixatives are alcohol-based, and, therefore, cytology specimens are typically suitable for nucleic acid extraction for molecular assays [17, 23, 24]. However, alcohol is not a favored fixative in routine histology laboratories. Implementing IHC assays – originally standardized and validated on FFPE histologic tissue – for use with cytologic specimens requires a rigorous validation process. One study using effusion-based IHC for EGFR mutation detection demonstrated a sensitivity of 70–80% compared to RNA analysis from effusion cell pellets [25]. Another review evaluating ALK IHC performed on cytology samples, including smears, cytospins, and LBC preparations, found slightly lower sensitivity. This suggests that IHC assays performed on non-FFPE substrates may require additional optimization [22]. Furthermore, interpreting IHC and fluorescence in situ hybridization (FISH) on a cytology smear can be more challenging compared to standard FFPE tissue sections.

In clinical practice, the integration of pleural effusion cytology-based mutation testing has improved diagnostic yield and patient convenience. Despite its utility, meticulous technical execution and thorough validation remain essential to ensure reliable results.

4. Pleural effusion cell block

Pleural effusion cell block preparations are the most commonly used cytologic-specimen preparation employed for ancillary testing in lung cancer. FFPE cell blocks of malignant effusions serve as a robust and convenient source of tumor DNA. Pleural effusion cell block preparation involves concentrating cellular material from pleural fluid in a cytology laboratory, which is then embedded in paraffin and processed similarly to a tissue biopsy to produce hematoxylin-eosin slides [26]. Pleural effusion cell block analysis significantly improves cytological diagnostic yield for malignancy [27]. The cell blocks are a perfect fit to bridge cytology and histopathology.

The main advantage of the cell block technique is that cells resemble those seen in histology. Apart from increased cellularity, better morphological details are obtained by the cell block method, which includes preservation of the architectural patterns and can be utilized for testing, such as IHC, FISH, or DNA/RNA extraction [11, 28]. DNA/RNA is extracted from pleural effusion cell block sections using protocols similar to other FFPE tissues. Typically, several unstained sections (e.g., 5–10 sections of 5 μm thickness) are cut and deparaffinized for nucleic acid extraction. Kits optimized for FFPE samples, which include deparaffinization, proteinase K digestion, and purification steps, can also be used to isolate DNA from cell blocks. Tumor-rich areas can be macro-dissected from the sections to improve tumor DNA yield if needed. Studies have shown that DNA extracted from pleural fluid cell blocks is of comparable quality to that from tissue biopsies, indicating sufficient DNA integrity for downstream molecular tests [29]. This allows cell block DNA to be used for PCR-based assays and NGS panels. Several studies have confirmed that the status of oncogenic driver genes detected in MPE cell blocks is consistent with that in tumor tissues [30–32].

A study compared EGFR mutation results between MPE cell blocks and tissue samples using a sensitive PCR assay (ARMS). The sensitivity of the cell block versus tissue was around 81.8%, with an overall mutation status concordance of 81% [31]. Another study that applied targeted NGS on both pleural effusion cell blocks and corresponding tissue found high concordance in mutations detected, indicating that essentially the same driver alterations were found in both sample types [29]. DNA quality index analysis showed that DNA extracted from cell blocks of pleural fluid was of similar quality compared to FFPE tissue blocks [29].

There are some drawbacks to using cell blocks in molecular diagnosis. Cell blocks often vary in quality, and inadequate cellularity is the most common reason for suboptimal results. Cell-block testing yields depend on tumor cell fraction – low cellularity can lead to false-negatives. If tumor content is below the detection threshold, key driver mutations or fusions may be missed. Besides, histiocytes, leukocytes, mesothelial cells, and other benign components may dominate the sample, masking or diluting tumor cells. If the proportion of these cells is significantly higher than that of malignant cells, molecular methods are likely to fail or give erroneous results due to the intermixing of benign and malignant DNA. A study demonstrated that the minimum absolute number of tumor cells required for reliable molecular results ranged from approximately 300 cells when tumor cells constituted less than 20% of nucleated cells, down to approximately 170 cells when tumor cells comprised more than 50% of the sample [33]. Overall cellularity and tumor percentage, rather than specimen volume, are of prime importance for determining the efficacy of pleural fluid cell blocks for molecular studies. Cell blocks with a tumor cell proportion of $<20\%$ may not be appropriate for molecular studies, and a repeat specimen should be considered [33, 34]. Moreover, cell blocks are FFPE. Nucleic acids extracted from formalin-fixed cell blocks are prone to degradation, which can lead to sequencing artifacts and potential false-negative or false-positive results in downstream molecular assays [35].

Generally speaking, when tumor cellularity is adequate, pleural effusion cell blocks can reliably mirror tissue biopsy results for both histological diagnosis and genomic profiling.

5. Pleural effusion cfDNA

Liquid biopsy involves the analysis of tumor-derived materials present in body fluids and has demonstrated promising results when applied to pleural fluid cfDNA. The cell-free supernatant of pleural fluid was often discarded; however, recent technological advancements have enabled its analysis for cfDNA. This supernatant contains cfDNA shed by tumor cells and other cells within the pleural space. Given the anatomical proximity of the pleural space to lung tumors and involved lymphatics, pleural effusions are often enriched with tumor-derived DNA fragments [36]. These cfDNA fragments can be isolated and analyzed using methods such as PCR or NGS.

Studies have demonstrated that pleural effusion supernatant contains higher concentrations of tumor-derived cfDNA compared to concurrent plasma samples and pleural effusion sediment cells [36, 37]. Mutant allele frequencies in pleural effusion cfDNA are comparable to those found in matched tumor tissue samples and are significantly higher than in pleural effusion cell sediment DNA or plasma cfDNA, reflecting an enriched fraction of tumor-derived DNA [37]. This abundant source of tumor DNA makes pleural effusion cfDNA particularly suitable for mutation testing [36]. Because cfDNA analysis is not limited by sample cellularity, it can identify tumor mutations even in cytology-negative or paucicellular specimens.

Tissue biopsy remains the gold standard for molecular diagnosis, but pleural effusion cfDNA shows performance close to tissue and, in some scenarios, even captures mutations that tissue missed. Accumulating evidence indicates that pleural effusion cfDNA is a highly accurate medium for detecting driver mutations, often approaching the accuracy of tissue biopsy and outperforming pleural effusion cytology and plasma cfDNA [38]. While EGFR mutations have the most extensive validation, other driver mutations, including gene fusions, can also be reliably detected in pleural effusion cfDNA using appropriate NGS platforms.

A meta-analysis of 15 studies compared EGFR mutation testing in pleural effusion samples with traditional tissue genotyping. Results indicated that cfDNA from pleural fluid supernatant provided superior performance compared to cell-pellet analysis of pleural effusion sediments [13]. In a separate study using droplet digital PCR, pleural or pericardial effusion-derived cfDNA achieved 97% sensitivity, 97% specificity, and 97% concordance with tissue genotyping for detecting sensitizing EGFR variants. Additionally, effusion cfDNA demonstrated greater sensitivity compared to plasma cfDNA for EGFR mutation detection (97% vs. 74%) [39]. A multicenter trial directly compared NGS of malignant pleural effusion cfDNA with standard tissue or cell-block testing, finding that cfDNA analysis identified EGFR, ALK, and ROS1 mutations in 64.1% of cases, compared to 51.3% for standard methods [40]. Furthermore, a prospective study demonstrated that pleural effusion cfDNA analyzed by NGS detected actionable mutations in 88% of patients, compared to 78% detection by pleural effusion cell-pellet Sanger sequencing [41].

Plasma cfDNA genotyping is substantially affected by variability in tumor DNA shedding into the bloodstream. Studies have reported negative plasma cfDNA test results in approximately 32%, 21.9%, and 3% of patients with M1a, M1b, and M1c disease, respectively, despite the presence of driver mutations [6]. This high false-negative rate remains a critical barrier to the widespread clinical use of plasma cfDNA analysis, particularly among patients with limited metastatic disease. In contrast, pleural fluid is anatomically close to the tumor environment and typically has a higher tumor DNA burden. Therefore, pleural effusion cfDNA represents an excellent alternative to plasma for identifying genetic mutations, especially in patients with M1a disease and limited metastasis [41]. Testing pleural effusion cfDNA at disease progression doubles the T790M detection rate compared to plasma, identifying T790M in 50% of effusion cfDNA samples versus approximately 20% in plasma samples [42]. Similarly, a study employing droplet digital PCR demonstrated significantly higher T790M detection in pleural fluid compared with matched blood samples (51% vs. 25%) among patients progressing on first-line EGFR tyrosine kinase inhibitors [39].

Incorporating pleural effusion cfDNA analysis into clinical practice yields several clear advantages. Obtaining pleural fluid via thoracentesis is less invasive than surgical or bronchoscopic biopsies. It thus spares patients from repeated invasive biopsies solely for genotyping. Rather than relying solely on a sometimes-scant tissue biopsy, clinicians can perform parallel or sequential testing on pleural fluid. The fluid can be processed quickly: centrifugation yields a supernatant for cfDNA extraction, which can then be analyzed by PCR or NGS for key mutations. This directly translates into more patients being eligible for targeted therapies. Thoracentesis can be repeated if the effusion reaccumulates, enabling monitoring of molecular changes over time. This makes pleural cfDNA an excellent tool for tracking resistance mechanisms or clonal evolution without invasive procedures.

Cytology or cell-block analyses rely on the presence of malignant cells in pleural effusions, limiting their diagnostic utility in paramalignant effusions. However, analyzing cfDNA from pleural fluid can overcome this limitation, as tumor DNA is often detectable even when cytology results are negative. In fact, one study reported nearly identical mutation detection rates in cytology-positive and cytology-negative pleural effusions (mutations identified in 99% and 100% of samples, respectively), along with similar maximal allelic fractions [43]. Another study observed that in cytology-negative effusions where tumor cells were absent, DNA from the cell sediment often failed to detect mutations, whereas cfDNA analysis still succeeded [37]. Even in hemorrhagic effusions, where tumor DNA can be diluted by abundant blood-derived DNA, cfDNA analysis remained far superior to cell-sediment analysis for mutation detection [37]. Paramalignant effusions are nearly as informative as overt malignant effusions when modern cfDNA techniques are applied.

Several limitations and unresolved questions persist regarding the use of pleural effusion cfDNA for molecular diagnostics. Detection sensitivity for gene fusions in cfDNA is generally lower than for point mutations or indels due to DNA fragmentation, the structural complexity of rearrangements, the absence of RNA expression data, and the inherent technical limitations of cfDNA assays. Currently, no studies have specifically evaluated the diagnostic yield of mutation detection using cfDNA in cytology-negative or paramalignant pleural effusions. Moreover, while plasma cfDNA protocols are relatively well-established in clinical laboratories, standardized approaches for analyzing pleural fluid cfDNA remain limited. Robust methods for handling large-volume fluids, effective DNA extraction protocols, and consistent assay performance are essential. Additionally, clonal hematopoiesis of indeterminate potential (CHIP) mutations can introduce background noise, increasing the risk of false-positive results and complicating the accurate interpretation of genuine somatic mutations in advanced NSCLC [44–47].

Pleural effusion cfDNA testing aligns with the goals of precision oncology by being sensitive, minimally invasive, and actionable – ensuring that treatable mutations are not missed and that patients receive the right therapies at the right time.

6. Emerging technique

In addition to DNA-based biomarkers, other liquid biopsy components are under investigation, including circulating tumor cells (CTCs), cell-free RNA (cfRNA), as well as exosomes and microRNAs. CTCs are highly tumor-specific; however, they are extremely rare in circulation and technically challenging to isolate reliably. As a result, CTCs are not yet utilized in routine clinical practice. By contrast, cfRNA is an emerging biomarker that shows promising potential for the molecular diagnosis of NSCLC.

Cancer cells can undergo cell death through apoptosis or necrosis, resulting in the passive release of circulating tumor DNA (ctDNA) into the bloodstream [48]. In addition to passive mechanisms, ctDNA can also be actively secreted via extracellular vesicles. The clinical utility of circulating tumor DNA/cell-free DNA (ctDNA/cfDNA) in molecular diagnosis for NSCLC has been well established. Meanwhile, circulating cell-free tumor RNA (ctRNA), comprising tumor-derived RNA molecules released into circulation, is predominantly released through active secretion mechanisms, as passive release typically results in rapid degradation [49]. Levels of cfRNA corresponding to classic solid tumor markers are significantly elevated in cancer patients, reflecting the abundant presence of circulating tumor-derived transcripts. This abundance facilitates their potential use in mutation detection assays [50]. Additionally, transcripts of mutated alleles often exceed their DNA fragment counterparts in plasma or effusion due to active gene expression, providing a biological amplification effect that enhances cfRNA as a promising analyte for robust mutation detection [50, 51].

Current evidence demonstrates that cfRNA analysis can detect a broad spectrum of driver mutations in NSCLC with high specificity, typically ranging between 90% and 100% [52, 53]. Properly designed assays rarely generate false positives. Sensitivity, however, varies across different study conditions. Notably, cfRNA has proven reliable for identifying EGFR mutations in NSCLC patients. When compared with cfDNA alone, a cfRNA-inclusive approach achieves superior sensitivity for detecting activating EGFR mutations (98% vs. 82%) and T790M mutations (90% vs. 84%) [54].

Moreover, cfRNA demonstrates superior performance over cfDNA for the detection of fusion genes and splice variants, potentially overcoming limitations associated with cfDNA analysis [50, 55]. Incorporating cfRNA into diagnostic testing notably enhances the identification of gene rearrangements, increasing detection rates by approximately 28.6% compared to cfDNA alone [56]. Combining cfRNA with cfDNA generally provides the highest diagnostic yield [56]. The advantages of including cfRNA are particularly significant in cases characterized by low tumor DNA burden or those limited to intrathoracic disease, with cfRNA analysis increasing mutation detection rates by two – to three-fold [54].

Overall, cfRNA is emerging as a valuable adjunct to current diagnostic strategies. Nevertheless, its clinical implementation for NSCLC genetic alteration detection remains limited due to the absence of standardized protocols, a lack of validated biomarker panels, and potential interference from non-cancer factors. Technical challenges such as cfRNA degradation, extraction inefficiencies, and detection limitations further constrain its reliability. Thus, advancements in analytic techniques and the identification of suitable reference genes will be crucial for the future integration of cfRNA into clinical practice.

7. Conclusions

Over the past decade, numerous global studies have established pleural effusion as a reliable source for molecular diagnostics in NSCLC. Adequately cellular pleural fluid is now nearly equivalent to small biopsy specimens as a substrate for molecular testing. Although cell block preparations remain beneficial when sufficient tumor cells are available, cfDNA analysis has effectively overcome the challenge of low cellularity. Compared to traditional cytology and small biopsies, pleural supernatant cfDNA achieves superior sensitivity and high concordance with tissue genotypes. Continued advances in sensitive molecular techniques are expected to further reinforce the role of liquid biopsy, cementing its position as an integral component of precision oncology in lung cancer management. However, careful attention to laboratory procedures and mutation panels remains essential to prevent false-negative results or missed genetic alterations.

Pleural effusion serves as a compelling liquid biopsy source, complementing plasma and tissue biopsies for comprehensive genotyping. Current evidence robustly supports the integration of pleural effusion molecular testing into the routine diagnostic evaluation of advanced NSCLC, improving driver mutation detection and informing personalized treatment strategies, ultimately translating into better outcomes in advanced lung cancer.

Conflict of interest

The authors declare no conflict of interest.

Author details

Hsin-Yi Wang[1] and Jin-Yuan Shih[2*]

1 National Taiwan University Cancer Centre, Taipei City, Taiwan

2 Department of Internal Medicine, National Taiwan University Hospital, Taipei City, Taiwan

*Address all correspondence to: shihjy@ntu.edu.tw

References

[1] Papiris SA, Roussos C. Clinical Presentation of Lung Cancer. In Syrigos KN, Nutting CM, Roussos C, editors. Tumors of the Chest: Biology, Diagnosis and Management. Berlin, Heidelberg: Springer Berlin Heidelberg; 2006. p. 109–120

[2] Management of malignant pleural effusions. American Journal of Respiratory and Critical Care Medicine. 2000, **162**, 1987–2001

[3] Lindeman NI, Cagle PT, Aisner DL, et al. Updated Molecular Testing Guideline for the Selection of Lung Cancer Patients for Treatment With Targeted Tyrosine Kinase Inhibitors: Guideline From the College of American Pathologists, the International Association for the Study of Lung Cancer, and the Association for Molecular Pathology. Archives of Pathology and Laboratory Medicine. 2018;**142**:321–346

[4] Riely GJ, Wood DE, Ettinger DS, et al. Non–Small Cell Lung Cancer, Version 4.2024, NCCN Clinical Practice Guidelines in Oncology. Journal of the National Comprehensive Cancer Network. 2024;**22**:249–274

[5] Aggarwal C, Thompson JC, Black TA, et al. Clinical Implications of plasma-based genotyping with the delivery of personalized therapy in metastatic non–small cell lung cancer. JAMA Oncology. 2019;**5**:173–180

[6] Wang H-Y, Ho -C-C, Lin Y-T, et al. Comprehensive genomic analysis of patients with non–small-cell lung cancer using blood-based circulating tumor DNA assay: Findings from the BFAST database of a single center in Taiwan. JCO Precision Oncology. 2024;**8**: e2300314

[7] Grigoriadou G I , Esagian SM, Ryu HS, Nikas IP. Molecular profiling of malignant pleural effusions with next generation sequencing (NGS): Evidence that supports its role in cancer management. Journal of Personalized Medicine. 2020;**10**:206

[8] Rolfo C, Mack P, Scagliotti GV, et al. Liquid biopsy for advanced NSCLC: A consensus statement from the international association for the study of lung cancer. Journal of Thoracic Oncology. 2021;**16**:1647–1662

[9] Hummelink K, Muller M, Linders TC, et al. Cell-free DNA in the supernatant of pleural effusion can be used to detect driver and resistance mutations, and can guide tyrosine kinase inhibitor treatment decisions. ERJ Open Research. 2019;**5**:00016–02019

[10] Steinfort DP, Kranz S, Dowers A, et al. Sensitive molecular testing methods can demonstrate NSCLC driver mutations in malignant pleural effusion despite non-malignant cytology. Translational Lung Cancer Research. 2019;**8**:513–518

[11] Roy-Chowdhuri S, Aisner DL, Allen TC, et al. Biomarker testing in lung carcinoma cytology specimens: A perspective from members of the pulmonary pathology society. Archives of Pathology and Laboratory Medicine. 2016;**140**:1267–1272

[12] Chan C, Chan KKP. Pleural fluid biomarkers: A narrative review. Journal of Thoracic Disease. 2024;**16**:4764–4771

[13] Pang C, Ma H, Qin J, et al. Pleural effusion as a substitute for tumor tissue in detecting EGFR/ALK mutations in non-small cell lung cancer: A systematic review and meta-analysis. Medicine. 2019;**98**(18):e15450

[14] Buttitta F, Felicioni L, Del Grammastro M, et al. Effective assessment of EGFR mutation status in bronchoalveolar lavage and pleural fluids by next-generation sequencing. Clinical Cancer Research. 2013;**19**:691–698

[15] Wu SG, Liu YN, Yu CJ, et al. Driver mutations of young lung adenocarcinoma patients with malignant pleural effusion. Genes, Chromosomes and Cancer. 2018;**57**:513–521

[16] Wu S-G, Gow C-H, Yu C-J, et al. Frequent epidermal growth factor receptor gene mutations in malignant pleural effusion of lung adenocarcinoma. European Respiratory Journal. 2008;**32**:924–930

[17] Lindeman NI, Cagle PT, Beasley MB, et al. Molecular testing guideline for selection of lung cancer patients for EGFR and ALK tyrosine kinase inhibitors: Guideline from the college of american pathologists, international association for the study of lung cancer, and association for molecular pathology. The Journal of Molecular Diagnostics: JMD. 2013;**15**:415–453

[18] Balla A, Hampel KJ, Sharma MK, et al. Comprehensive validation of cytology specimens for next-generation sequencing and clinical practice experience. The Journal of Molecular Diagnostics. 2018;**20**:812–821

[19] Williams C, Pontén F, Moberg C, et al. A high frequency of sequence alterations is due to formalin fixation of archival specimens. The American Journal of Pathology. 1999;**155**:1467–1471

[20] Nakashima K, Otsubo K, Tsuchiya-Kawano Y, et al. Suitability of frozen pleural fluid pellets for next-generation sequencing-based driver gene testing in non-small cell lung cancer. Thoracic Cancer. 2025;**16**:e70107

[21] Fujii T, Uchiyama T, Matsuoka M, et al. Evaluation of DNA and RNA quality from archival formalin-fixed paraffin-embedded tissue for next-generation sequencing - Retrospective study in Japanese single institution. Pathology International. 2020;**70**:602–611

[22] Roy-Chowdhuri S. Immunocytochemistry of cytology specimens for predictive biomarkers in lung cancer. Translational Lung Cancer Research. 2020;**9**:898–905

[23] Malapelle U, Bellevicine C, Zeppa P, et al. Cytology-based gene mutation tests to predict response to anti-epidermal growth factor receptor therapy: A review. Diagnostic Cytopathology. 2011;**39**:703–710

[24] Aisner DL, Deshpande C, Baloch Z, et al. Evaluation of EGFR mutation status in cytology specimens: An institutional experience. Diagnostic Cytopathology. 2013;**41**:316–323

[25] Tsai TH, Wu SG, Chang YL, et al. Effusion immunocytochemistry as an alternative approach for the selection of first-line targeted therapy in advanced lung adenocarcinoma. Journal of Thoracic Oncology. 2012;**7**:993–1000

[26] Saqi A. The state of cell blocks and ancillary testing: Past, present, and future. Archives of Pathology and Laboratory Medicine. 2016;**140**:1318–1322

[27] Assawasaksakul T, Boonsarngsuk V, Incharoen P. A comparative study of conventional cytology and cell block method in the diagnosis of pleural effusion. Journal of Thoracic Disease. 2017;**9**:3161–3167

[28] Ugurluoglu C, Kurtipek E, Unlu Y, et al. Importance of the cell block technique in diagnosing patients with non-small cell carcinoma accompanied by pleural effusion. Asian Pacific Journal of Cancer Prevention. 2015;**16**:3057–3060

[29] Zhang Y, Li J, Hua P, et al. Targeted next-generation sequencing in cytology specimens for molecular profiling of lung adenocarcinoma. International Journal of Clinical and Experimental Pathology. 2018;**11**:3647–3655

[30] Lin R, Li Y, Lin Y, et al. Role of molecular testing for malignant pleural effusion in targeted therapy for advanced non-small cell lung cancer. Diagnostic Cytopathology. 2023;**51**:397–405

[31] Liu X, Lu Y, Zhu G, et al. The diagnostic accuracy of pleural effusion and plasma samples versus tumour tissue for detection of EGFR mutation in patients with advanced non-small cell lung cancer: Comparison of methodologies. Journal of Clinical Pathology. 2013;**66**:1065–1069

[32] Liu N, Sun RZ, Du J, et al. Comparison of epidermal growth factor receptor gene mutations identified using pleural effusion and primary tumor tissue samples in non-small cell lung cancer. Applied Immunohistochemistry and Molecular Morphology. 2018;**26**:e44–e51

[33] Dalvi SD, Chau K, Sajjan S, et al. Adequacy of pleural fluid cytology for comprehensive molecular analysis of lung adenocarcinoma: Experience of a large health-care system. Cytojournal. 2022;**19**:7

[34] Akca Y, Erkilic S. Methodological and TNM focus-based comparison of egfr mutation status in non-small-cell lung carcinomas. Journal of Cytology. 2024;**41**:171–175

[35] Bellevicine C, Malapelle U, de Luca C, et al. EGFR analysis: Current evidence and future directions. Diagnostic Cytopathology. 2014;**42**:984–992

[36] Mokánszki A, Bádon ES, Mónus A, et al. Cell-free DNA from pleural effusion samples: is it right for molecular testing in lung adenocarcinoma? Pathology & Oncology Research. 2021;**27**:613071.

[37] Tong L, Ding N, Tong X, et al. Tumor-derived DNA from pleural effusion supernatant as a promising alternative to tumor tissue in genomic profiling of advanced lung cancer. Theranostics. 2019;**9**:5532–5541

[38] Mahmood K, Jampani P, Clarke JM, et al. High yield of pleural cell-free DNA for diagnosis of oncogenic mutations in lung adenocarcinoma. Chest. 2023;**164**:252–261

[39] Lee KWC, Msc L, Gai W, et al. Testing for EGFR variants in pleural and pericardial effusion cell-free DNA in patients with non–small cell lung cancer. JAMA Oncology. 2023;**9**:261–265

[40] Chang SC, Wei YF, Chen CY, et al. Profiling cell-free DNA from malignant pleural effusion for oncogenic driver mutations in patients with treatment-naive stage IV adenocarcinoma: A multicenter prospective study. Molecular Diagnosis & Therapy. 2024;**28**(6):803–810

[41] Wang HY, Liao W-Y, Ho CC, et al. Enhanced detection of actionable mutations in NSCLC through pleural effusion cell-free DNA sequencing: A prospective study. European Journal of Cancer. 2025;**217**:115224

[42] Vukovic M, Tanic M, Damjanovic A, et al. EGFR mutation testing from pleural effusions of non-small cell lung cancer patients at the institute for oncology and radiology of Serbia. Translational Oncology. 2023;**37**:101772.

[43] Song Z, Wang W, Li M, et al. Cytological-negative pleural effusion can be an alternative liquid biopsy media for detection of EGFR mutation in NSCLC patients. Lung Cancer: Targets and Therapy. 2019;**136**:23–29

[44] Hu Y, Ulrich BC, Supplee J, et al. False-positive plasma genotyping due to clonal hematopoiesis. Clinical Cancer Research. 2018;**24**:4437–4443

[45] Ptashkin RN, Mandelker DL, Coombs CC, et al. Prevalence of clonal hematopoiesis mutations in tumor-only clinical genomic profiling of solid tumors. JAMA Oncology. 2018;**4**:1589–1593

[46] Yaung SJ, Fuhlbrück F, Peterson M, et al. Clonal hematopoiesis in late-stage non-small-cell lung cancer and its impact on targeted panel next-generation sequencing. JCO Precision Oncology. 2020;**4**:1271–1279

[47] Yang X, Wang Y, Li Y, et al. Clonal hematopoiesis in lung cancer and its impact on liquid biopsy based on targeted deep sequencing. Journal of Clinical Oncology. 2022;**40**:e20532–e20532

[48] Schwarzenbach H, Hoon DSB, Pantel K. Cell-free nucleic acids as biomarkers in cancer patients. Nature Reviews Cancer. 2011;**11**:426–437

[49] Stejskal P, Goodarzi H, Srovnal J, et al. Circulating tumor nucleic acids: Biology, release mechanisms, and clinical relevance. Molecular Cancer. 2023;**22**:15

[50] Albitar M, Zhang H, Charifa A, et al. Combining cell-free RNA with cell-free DNA in liquid biopsy for hematologic and solid tumors. Heliyon. 2023;**9**:e16261

[51] Tsai TH, Su KY, Wu SG, et al. RNA is favourable for analysing EGFR mutations in malignant pleural effusion of lung cancer. European Respiratory Journal. 2012;**39**:677–684

[52] Heeke S, Benzaquen J, Vallee A, et al. Detection of ALK fusion transcripts in plasma of non-small cell lung cancer patients using a novel RT-PCR based assay. Annals of Translational Medicine. 2021;**9**:922

[53] Kim Y, Shin S, Lee K-A. Exosome-based detection of EGFR T790M in plasma and pleural fluid of prospectively enrolled non-small cell lung cancer patients after first-line tyrosine kinase inhibitor therapy. Cancer Cell International. 2021;**21**:50

[54] Lazzari C, Gregorc V, Cangi MG, et al. Combined exosomal RNA and circulating tumor DNA for epidermal growth factor mutation detection in non-small cell lung cancer. Journal of Thoracic Disease. 2018;**10**:S4023–S4027

[55] Hasegawa N, Kohsaka S, Kurokawa K, et al. Highly sensitive fusion detection using plasma cell-free RNA in non-small-cell lung cancers. Cancer Science. 2021;**112**:4393–4403

[56] Samol J, Ng D, Poh J, et al. Prospective multicenter study evaluating a combined circulating tumor DNA and circulating tumor RNA liquid biopsy in metastatic non-small cell lung cancer (LIQUIK). JCO Precision Oncology. 2025;**9**:e2500181

Chapter 7

Pleural Biomarkers in Diagnosis and Prognosis: Current Evidence and Clinical Applications

Fatma Selen Ala Çitlak

Abstract

Pleural fluid analysis remains a cornerstone in the differential diagnosis of pleural effusions. In recent years, the identification and utilization of pleural biomarkers have significantly advanced diagnostic accuracy and prognostic stratification in various pleural diseases. From malignancies such as malignant pleural effusion (MPE) to infectious causes like parapneumonic effusions, and transudative processes including heart failure, specific biomarkers offer valuable insight into disease etiology, activity, and progression. Biomarkers such as mesothelin, fibulin-3, NT-proBNP, and procalcitonin have shown promising results in distinguishing between benign and malignant effusions, predicting treatment outcomes, and reducing the need for invasive procedures. This chapter reviews recent findings from the 2024 literature, highlighting key biomarkers, their mechanisms, diagnostic thresholds, and their integration into clinical practice. The goal is to provide a practical and evidence-based overview of how pleural biomarkers contribute to improved decision-making and patient care in pleural disease management.

Keywords: pleural effusion, exudative effusion, transudative effusion, pleural biomarkers, pleural fluid analysis

1. Introduction

Pleural fluid analysis remains a cornerstone in the differential diagnosis of pleural effusions. While Light's criteria are widely accepted and have been used for decades to differentiate between transudative and exudative effusions, they often fall short in identifying the underlying etiology. Despite their longevity, Light's criteria continue to be the first step in evaluating pleural effusions. However, concerns persist regarding their diagnostic accuracy. For instance, although Light's criteria are highly sensitive in distinguishing transudates from exudates, they misclassify approximately 20–30% of transudative effusions due to congestive heart failure or cirrhosis as exudates, particularly in patients undergoing diuretic therapy [1].

Studies have shown that most of these false exudate diagnoses occur in patients receiving diuretics, which can alter serum and pleural fluid biochemical parameters [2].

This raises the question of whether evaluating effusions based solely on biochemical parameters is sufficient or clinically meaningful. Moreover, in cases where clinical assessments do not align with laboratory results, a re-evaluation of diagnostic priorities may be necessary. It is also important to consider that certain etiologies can result in both transudative and exudative effusions, and, in rare instances, both types may coexist in a single patient.

In such complex scenarios, where the distinction between transudate and exudate is unclear, clinical findings and the patient's overall status should take precedence over biochemical tests in guiding diagnostic decisions. Additionally, an important challenge lies in the determination of threshold levels for biochemical parameters, as the sensitivity and specificity of any diagnostic test depend on the defined cut-off values. Incorrect thresholds can lead to false-positive or false-negative results, undermining diagnostic reliability.

Therefore, the demand for more accurate, rapid, and non-invasive diagnostic methods has increased in recent years. Biomarkers have emerged as promising, targeted, and molecular-based tools capable of addressing this diagnostic gap. These biomarkers provide essential diagnostic and prognostic information in a variety of pleural effusion etiologies, including malignancies (e.g., malignant pleural effusion [MPE]), infectious diseases (e.g., tuberculosis, parapneumonic effusions), and systemic conditions such as heart failure.

Biomarkers may also reduce the need for invasive diagnostic procedures by enabling more precise identification of the fluid's origin and allowing for earlier therapeutic intervention. For example, in exudative effusions, novel biomarkers are required to enable early etiological classification without the need for invasive diagnostic procedures (e.g., pleural biopsy, thoracoscopy) or therapeutic procedures (e.g., repeated thoracenteses, chest tube insertion). Prominent candidates that have demonstrated promise in differentiating between malignant and infectious etiologies include mesothelin, fibulin-3, N-terminal pro-B-type natriuretic peptide (NT-proBNP), procalcitonin (PCT), adenosine deaminase (ADA), and carcinoembryonic antigen (CEA) [3].

In the 2020s, biomarker research has expanded beyond traditional protein-based markers to include emerging technologies such as exosomes, microRNAs, metabolomics, and proteomics approaches [4]. Despite these advancements, clinical integration remains limited due to analytical variability, lack of standardization, and uncertain cut-off values [5].

This book chapter aims to provide a systematic evaluation of the diagnostic and prognostic utility of pleural biomarkers based on the latest literature. It addresses key aspects such as specificity, sensitivity, diagnostic thresholds, biological mechanisms, and clinical integration strategies. The overarching goal is to present a practical, evidence-based overview of how pleural biomarkers can enhance clinical decision-making in pleural disease management and make recent developments more accessible to healthcare professionals.

2. Classification of pleural biomarkers

Pleural biomarkers can be classified based on their clinical function, biological origin, and etiological relevance. This classification provides a structured framework for research and facilitates the integration of biomarkers into clinical practice.

2.1. Classification by clinical function

Diagnostic biomarkers: These are used to confirm or exclude the presence of a disease. For instance, ADA is commonly used for diagnosing tuberculous pleural effusion (TPE), while NT-proBNP is useful for identifying pleural effusions secondary to heart failure [6, 7].

Prognostic biomarkers: These biomarkers help predict disease progression, mortality risk, or response to therapy. For example, mesothelin levels in MPEs can provide prognostic insights [8].

Therapeutic decision-making biomarkers: These markers guide treatment decisions, particularly in infectious effusions. For instance, PCT levels can influence the initiation or discontinuation of antibiotic therapy [9].

2.2. Classification by biological source

Systemically derived biomarkers: These include markers such as NT-proBNP and C-reactive protein (CRP), which typically diffuse from the serum into the pleural space.

Locally produced biomarkers: Biomarkers such as ADA, mesothelin, and fibulin-3 are secreted by local mesothelial, inflammatory, or tumor cells.

Extracellular vesicle/exosome-based biomarkers: In recent years, exosomes carrying microRNAs and protein complexes have gained attention as diagnostic tools [4].

2.3. Classification by etiological association

Malignancy-associated biomarkers: Examples include mesothelin, fibulin-3, CEA, Cancer Antigen (CA) 15-3, and CYFRA 21-1.

Infection-associated biomarkers: These include ADA, interferon-gamma (IFN-γ), CRP, IL-6, and PCT.

Transudative effusion-associated biomarkers: NT-proBNP, serum-pleural albumin gradient, chloride gradient, and novel cardiac biomarkers are commonly associated.

This structured classification facilitates the development of diagnostic algorithms and allows clinicians to contextualize the significance of each biomarker. In particular, combining multiple biomarkers within diagnostic protocols enhances both sensitivity and specificity, resulting in more reliable clinical outcomes [10].

3. Exudative pleural effusions

Exudative pleural effusions result from increased pleural membrane permeability, impaired lymphatic drainage, or protein leakage due to inflammation. The most common causes include malignancy, tuberculosis, pneumonia/parapneumonic effusions, pulmonary embolism, autoimmune diseases, and pancreatitis. Diagnostic challenges are especially pronounced in differentiating between malignant and infectious causes.

3.1. Malignant pleural effusions (MPEs)

MPE is one of the most frequent causes of exudative effusion. MPE typically arises from metastatic involvement of the pleura via lymphatic or hematogenous spread. Tumor-secreted vascular endothelial growth factor (VEGF) contributes to increased capillary permeability, while lymphatic obstruction represents a secondary mechanism.

Primary cancers leading to MPE include those of the lung, breast, genitourinary tract (especially the ovary), gastrointestinal tract, and lymphomas. Asbestos exposure is a known risk factor for malignant mesothelioma, another important cause of MPE. The presence of MPE often indicates advanced disease and is associated with a poor prognosis. Median survival ranges between 4 and 12 months, with the shortest survival in lung cancer and the longest in ovarian cancer.

The diagnosis is established through the detection of malignant cells in pleural fluid. While cytology, pleural biopsy, and imaging techniques are standard, pleural fluid cytology has a limited sensitivity of 60–70% [11]. The diagnostic yield is lower in squamous cell carcinoma and lymphoma compared to adenocarcinoma. Cytology confirms only one-third of mesothelioma cases.

To differentiate MPE from benign effusions, tumor markers must demonstrate cut-off values below which all benign effusions fall, thus achieving 100% specificity, albeit at the expense of sensitivity. Consequently, non-invasive biomarkers are crucial for diagnosing MPE and identifying the underlying malignancy.

Numerous studies have explored the diagnostic and prognostic roles of tumor markers in pleural effusions, including CEA, alpha-fetoprotein (AFP), p53, CA 15-3, CA 19-9, CA 72-4, CA 549, CYFRA 21-1, CA 125, neuron-specific enolase (NSE), mesothelin, squamous cell carcinoma antigen (SCC), HER-2/neu, fibronectin, TSA, and telomerase [12,13].

In the following sections, we will review the most relevant and commonly studied pleural biomarkers in the context of malignancy.

3.2. Mesothelin

Mesothelin is a 40 kDa glycoprotein tethered to the mesothelial cell membrane via phosphatidylinositol. Elevated mesothelin levels in pleural fluid suggest malignancy, particularly mesothelioma and adenocarcinoma. Numerous studies have examined its diagnostic value in mesothelioma, consistently demonstrating statistically significant increases in mesothelin levels in MPEs compared to benign effusions. Although sensitivity is modest (~65%), specificity reaches approximately 90%, indicating high diagnostic value [14,15].

Davies et al. proposed an optimal cutoff value of 20 nM for pleural mesothelin, yielding an AUC of 0.878, a sensitivity of 71%, and a specificity of 90% for differentiating mesothelioma from other MPEs and benign effusions [16]. However, elevated mesothelin levels may also occur in lung adenocarcinoma, limiting its standalone diagnostic utility. While mesothelin appears to be a promising biomarker for mesothelioma, histopathological confirmation remains the gold standard.

3.3. Fibulin-3

Fibulin-3 is an extracellular matrix glycoprotein involved in cell adhesion, proliferation, and angiogenesis. Its levels are elevated in both malignant mesothelioma and other metastatic solid tumors. Particularly in mesothelioma, fibulin-3 has demonstrated strong diagnostic performance in pleural fluid [17].

In a study by Creaney et al. involving 153 patients (82 with mesothelioma, 36 with non-mesothelioma MPE, and 35 with benign effusions), mesothelin outperformed fibulin-3 in both plasma (AUC 0.822 vs. 0.671) and pleural fluid (AUC 0.815 vs. 0.588) [18]. Despite its lower diagnostic value compared to mesothelin, pleural fluid fibulin-3 has emerged as an independent prognostic marker. When used in combination with mesothelin, fibulin-3 can enhance diagnostic sensitivity [19]. It is unaffected by age, sex, or body mass index and demonstrates high specificity.

3.4. Carcinoembryonic antigen (CEA)

CEA is a non-specific tumor marker often elevated in lung and gastrointestinal adenocarcinomas. It is commonly used to differentiate benign from MPEs but is less effective in diagnosing mesothelioma. CEA levels above 5 ng/mL in pleural fluid suggest malignancy [20].

A meta-analysis of 45 studies involving 2,834 MPE and 3,251 non-MPE cases reported a sensitivity of 54%, a specificity of 94%, and an AUC of 0.86 for CEA [21]. High levels of CEA in adenocarcinomas reduce its predictive value for mesothelioma. Therefore, a high CEA level in pleural fluid effectively rules out mesothelioma and is particularly useful for distinguishing between mesothelioma and metastatic lung cancer.

3.5. CA 15-3 and CYFRA 21-1

CA 15-3, a glycoprotein product of the MUC-1 gene, is a non-specific tumor marker also found in serum. It is particularly useful in diagnosing MPE associated with breast cancer. Its sensitivity and specificity in distinguishing malignant from benign effusions have been reported as 80% and 93%, respectively [22].

CYFRA 21-1, also known as cytokeratin 19 fragment, is a cytoplasmic protein released from tumor cells. It is especially useful in squamous cell lung carcinoma. CYFRA 21-1 demonstrates over 90% sensitivity and specificity in differentiating malignant from benign effusions. When used in combination, CA 15-3 and CYFRA 21-1 improve diagnostic accuracy [23].

3.6. Survivin

Survivin is a 16.5 kDa protein that inhibits apoptosis and plays a role in cancer development. As a novel biomarker, survivin is involved in diagnosis, prognosis, and predicting response to cancer therapy. Overexpression of survivin is associated with poor prognosis and resistance to chemotherapy or radiotherapy. Several studies have examined its role in the diagnosis and prognosis of MPE. Elevated survivin levels or mRNA expression in pleural fluid are linked to decreased survival and can distinguish between favorable and unfavorable prognostic groups [24].

3.7. Vascular endothelial growth factor (VEGF)

VEGF-A is a key cytokine involved in the pathogenesis of MPE. Produced by tumor cells, mesothelial cells, and infiltrating immune cells, high VEGF levels promote vascular permeability, tumor cell migration, and angiogenesis. Elevated VEGF levels are found in both malignant and benign pleural effusions, although they are consistently higher in malignant effusions [25].

VEGF detection in pleural fluid may aid in MPE diagnosis, but its standalone diagnostic value is limited [26]. VEGF levels above 2,000 pg/mL in malignant mesothelioma are associated with poor prognosis [27]. Intrathoracic anti-VEGF therapies are being investigated as a potential treatment for MPE [28].

3.8. Combined use of biomarkers

Because no single biomarker offers sufficient sensitivity and specificity, combining multiple biomarkers is often recommended. For instance, combining mesothelin with CEA improves both specificity and positive predictive value [29].

Effective clinical application of these biomarkers requires proper patient selection, defined cutoff values, and technical standardization. Furthermore, improved understanding of the biology underlying malignant effusions may guide therapeutic strategies.

4. Infectious pleural effusions and biomarkers

Infectious pleural effusions – including parapneumonic effusions, empyema, and tuberculous pleurisy – are commonly encountered and present significant diagnostic challenges. Distinguishing between bacterial and mycobacterial etiologies is essential for guiding treatment and determining the need for invasive interventions. In these cases, biomarkers play a critical role in accelerating diagnosis, targeting empirical therapy, and minimizing unnecessary procedures.

4.1. Adenosine deaminase (ADA)

Pathophysiology and role: ADA is an enzyme involved in purine catabolism, converting adenosine to inosine and deoxyadenosine to deoxyinosine. It is predominantly found in T lymphocytes, where it plays a critical role in cellular differentiation and immune activity. Due to the cell-mediated immune response characteristic of TPE, ADA levels are significantly elevated in this condition. ADA is a rapid, inexpensive, and easily repeatable test. A pleural ADA level >40 IU/L is considered diagnostically significant, especially in regions with a high prevalence of tuberculosis [30]. In such areas, the presence of elevated pleural ADA in lymphocyte-predominant exudates (usually >40 IU/L) is often sufficient to initiate empirical anti-tuberculosis therapy (ATT) [31].

Meta-analyses report a sensitivity of approximately 92% and a specificity of about 90% for ADA in diagnosing TPE [32]. In young patients and in lymphocyte-dominant effusions, ADA levels >70 IU/L are considered highly indicative of tuberculosis. Tay and Tee identified a significant negative correlation between ADA activity and age ($r = -0.621$), suggesting that lower ADA cutoffs should be considered in elderly patients (>55 years) with suspected TPE. Very high ADA activity (>250 IU/L) may suggest empyema or lymphoma. However, elevated ADA levels can also be seen in lymphomas and rheumatoid pleuritis. ADA elevation has also been reported in other malignancies (e.g., lymphoma, bronchoalveolar carcinoma, mesothelioma), infectious diseases (e.g., Mycoplasma and Chlamydia pneumoniae, psittacosis, paragonimiasis, infectious mononucleosis, brucellosis, histoplasmosis), and connective tissue diseases (e.g., rheumatoid arthritis, systemic lupus erythematosus) [33].

Given its affordability, speed, simplicity, reproducibility, and reliability, ADA is considered an ideal biomarker for diagnosing TPE.

Clinical case example:

A 35-year-old patient presented with fever, weight loss, and unilateral pleural effusion. Pleural ADA was measured at 85 IU/L, with a lymphocyte predominance of 95%. ATT was initiated prior to culture results based on these findings.

4.2. Interferon-gamma (IFN-γ) and other cytokines

Pathophysiology and diagnostic role: IFN-γ is a cytokine secreted by CD4 + T lymphocytes in tuberculous pleuritis, playing a key role in macrophage activation and antimicrobial defense. There are two primary methods for assessing IFN-γ levels in pleural effusions. The first is direct quantification of IFN-γ concentration in the pleural fluid. The second involves stimulation of sensitized T lymphocytes in the pleural effusion with Mycobacterium tuberculosis-specific antigens, such as culture filtrate protein-10 (CFP-10) and early secretory antigen-6 (ESAT-6), subsequently measuring released IFN-γ (as in the QuantiFERON-TB Gold test) or the number of IFN-γ-secreting T cells (as in the T-SPOT.TB test). These latter methods are known as IFN-γ release assays (IGRAs) [33].

Limitations and comparative value: A major limitation of direct IFN-γ testing is the absence of universally accepted cutoff values and the high associated costs. Despite these limitations, IFN-γ has demonstrated comparable diagnostic performance to ADA, particularly in high tuberculosis-burden settings.

The combination of IFN-γ and ADA testing has shown enhanced diagnostic performance. One meta-analysis involving 782 patients with TPE and 1,319 patients with non-TPE causes of pleural effusion reported that IFN-γ alone had a sensitivity of 89% and specificity of 97%. When used in combination with ADA, the sensitivity and specificity increased to 95% [34]. Although IFN-γ may offer slightly higher diagnostic accuracy, ADA remains more widely used due to its cost-effectiveness and ease of use in clinical settings [35].

Combined use: Studies evaluating both ADA and IFN-γ levels in pleural fluid have reported sensitivities and specificities exceeding 93%, with IFN-γ achieving specificity up to 96% (range: 94–97%) compared to ADA's 90–91%. The use of both markers in tandem enhances diagnostic reliability, particularly in ambiguous cases [36].

Interleukin-27 (IL-27): IL-27, a member of the IL-12 cytokine family produced by activated antigen-presenting cells, has emerged as a promising biomarker for TPE. It promotes CD4 + T cell proliferation and Th1 immune responses. IL-27 levels correlate with IFN-γ and ADA levels and have demonstrated high diagnostic accuracy in distinguishing TPE from non-TPE causes, with sensitivity and specificity exceeding 93% and 97%, respectively [37, 38].

IP-10 (CXCL10): This IFN-γ-induced chemokine has shown promise as a supplementary diagnostic marker for TPE. Although its specificity is suboptimal, IP-10 may serve as a valuable exclusion tool in clinical practice [39].

Interleukin-8 (IL-8): IL-8 is a pro-inflammatory cytokine involved in neutrophil chemotaxis and is elevated in infectious parapneumonic effusions and empyema. A cutoff of ≥1,000 pg/mL has demonstrated sensitivity and specificity of 84% and 82%, respectively (AUC 0.87). When combined with CRP measurements, diagnostic accuracy for complicated parapneumonic effusions improves further [40].

4.3. Procalcitonin (PCT)

PCT is the prohormone of calcitonin and serves as a valuable inflammatory biomarker that increases specifically in bacterial infections. It is secreted primarily by the parafollicular C cells of the thyroid in response to proinflammatory stimuli of bacterial origin, unlike CRP, which can increase in various inflammatory states, including viral infections. In contrast, PCT levels typically remain low in viral infections and tuberculosis, offering diagnostic specificity [41].

In the context of pleural effusions, elevated PCT levels suggest bacterial involvement, such as empyema or complicated parapneumonic effusions. A serum PCT threshold > 0.5 ng/mL is considered supportive of bacterial parapneumonic effusion. Although studies on pleural PCT concentrations remain limited, increasing evidence indicates that pleural PCT also holds diagnostic promise. A meta-analysis has demonstrated that, at a cut-off value of 0.16 ng/mL, pleural PCT exhibits a sensitivity of 81.5% and a specificity of 72.1% [42]. Additionally, a Turkish study revealed that using a pleural PCT threshold of 0.285 ng/mL provides a specificity of 96.9%, albeit with a lower sensitivity of 66.6%, for diagnosing parapneumonic pleural effusions (PPPE) [43]. These findings indicate that PCT levels can aid in guiding antibiotic therapy initiation and determining its duration.

4.4. C-reactive protein (CRP) and leukocyte count

CRP is a hepatic acute-phase reactant that rises in response to inflammation and infection. In pleural effusions, particularly those of parapneumonic origin, CRP levels are significantly elevated compared to transudative or non-infectious exudative effusions [44]. A pleural neutrophil count exceeding 50% typically reflects an acute bacterial infection. When combined with CRP measurements, the total neutrophil count improves diagnostic specificity [45].

In clinical practice, a pleural CRP level >40 mg/L is indicative of a complicated parapneumonic effusion, as supported by several studies [46]. Recent evidence further suggests that while CRP demonstrates moderate diagnostic utility in identifying PPPE, the addition of PCT does not enhance diagnostic accuracy significantly [47]. Consequently, CRP is currently the preferred biomarker for diagnosing PPE.

However, clinicians should recognize the limitations of CRP. Being a non-specific marker, it can be elevated in systemic inflammatory conditions unrelated to pleural infections. Furthermore, the diagnostic performance of biomarkers in pleural fluid may be compromised by the lack of standardized laboratory methods and the temporal variability of cytokine expression. Many cytokines are prone to rapid degradation, potentially leading to underestimation or misinterpretation of the inflammatory status in the pleural space.

5. Transudative pleural effusions

Transudative pleural effusions (TrPEs) result from the filtration of fluid secondary to hydrostatic and/or oncotic pressure imbalances across intact pulmonary, portal, hepatic, systemic vasculature, or other compartments such as the renal collecting system or subarachnoid space. The most common cause is congestive heart failure, which facilitates the passage of interstitial fluid from the visceral pleura into the pleural cavity. These effusions are generally systemic in origin and may also be due to conditions such as nephrotic syndrome, cirrhosis, and peritoneal dialysis. These conditions lead to fluid leakage via elevated capillary pressures or reduced oncotic pressure across pleural membranes.

Light's criteria remain widely used in clinical practice to differentiate between transudative and exudative pleural effusions. However, in patients with heart failure receiving diuretic therapy, especially when the effusion appears hemorrhagic, more than 25% of TrPEs may be misclassified as exudates [48]. Consequently, the application of protein and albumin gradients has improved classification accuracy in diuretic-treated patients. A pleural effusion is expected to be transudative if the serum-pleural albumin gradient exceeds 1.2 g/dL or the serum-pleural protein gradient exceeds 3.1 g/dL. Still, in patients on diuretics, the effusion may be falsely identified as an exudate.

In routine practice, because protein levels are often measured initially for Light's criteria, it is recommended to first calculate the protein gradient. If results remain inconclusive, the albumin gradient should then be assessed. Alternatively, measuring NT-proBNP may also be informative.

NT-proBNP, albumin gradient, chloride gradient, and other novel cardiac biomarkers offer valuable diagnostic and prognostic insights for these effusions.

NT-proBNP: Brain natriuretic peptide (BNP) is a 108-amino-acid precursor synthesized by cardiomyocytes in response to increased pressure or volume load. Upon stimulation, this precursor (pro-BNP) is enzymatically cleaved into the biologically inactive 76-amino-acid N-terminal fragment (NT-proBNP) and the active 32-amino-acid BNP hormone. In the diagnostic evaluation of heart failure, serum BNP levels <100 pg/mL or NT-proBNP <300 pg/mL suggest that heart failure is unlikely. Conversely, serum BNP >of 500 pg/mL or NT-proBNP levels between 450 and 1,800 pg/mL (age-dependent) support a diagnosis of heart failure.

Porcel et al. [49] first reported elevated NT-proBNP levels in pleural effusions secondary to heart failure in 2004. Subsequent studies confirmed that NT-proBNP levels in pleural fluid are useful in diagnosing heart failure-related pleural effusions [50]. One study demonstrated that a cut-off of 2,200 pg/mL provided high sensitivity (89%) and moderate specificity (73%) for identifying such effusions [51].

Soluble ST2 (sST2) and interleukin-33 (IL-33): ST2 is an alarmin expressed abundantly at barrier sites and is involved in immune regulation and tissue homeostasis through the suppression of the tumorigenesis-2 receptor. IL-33 and its decoy receptor sST2 have been implicated in various pulmonary diseases, although they are rarely studied in pleural pathology. Recent research has linked sST2 to heart failure prognosis, potentially independent of NT-proBNP. Its role in pleural fluid is under investigation [52].

A study measuring IL-33 and sST2 levels in TrPE, MPE, and PPE) reported similar values across these categories. However, in TrPE, IL-33 and sST2 levels correlated significantly with lymphocyte count and lactate dehydrogenase (LDH), while in MPE, IL-33 correlated with sST2 and red blood cell count [53].

6. Parapneumonic and empyemic effusions

PCT, CRP, IL-6, IL-8: These biomarkers are instrumental in identifying the infectious nature of parapneumonic effusions. CRP is an acute-phase reactant synthesized by hepatocytes, with its production upregulated during infections and inflammatory processes. Alongside classical pleural fluid parameters, CRP is used to stratify patients into those with complicated or uncomplicated parapneumonic effusions. In contrast, PCT levels rise specifically in bacterial infections. However, few studies have evaluated these markers, and the existing literature suffers from limited sample sizes [54]. Elevated IL-6 and IL-8 levels are indicative of neutrophil activation and chemotaxis, as neutrophils are the predominant leukocyte population found in pleural fluid during acute inflammation. Studies have demonstrated that these cytokines can distinguish between empyema and complicated parapneumonic effusions [55].

Macrophage migration inhibitory factor (MIF): MIF plays a regulatory role in inflammatory immune responses and is produced by various immune cells. It is significantly elevated in conditions such as complicated parapneumonic pleural effusion (CPPE) and empyema [56].

IL-1β, IL-36γ, MIP-3α: These cytokines have been found in high concentrations in empyemic cases and may serve as diagnostic markers for differentiating severe infectious effusions [57].

6.1. Autoimmune-related effusions

Antinuclear antibody (ANA), rheumatoid factor (RF), Anti-dsDNA: In lupus or rheumatoid arthritis-related pleural involvement, these autoantibodies are more diagnostically significant in pleural fluid than in serum. ANA has demonstrated adequate sensitivity and specificity for differentiating lupus pleuritis from other etiologies of pleural effusion [58].

7. Emerging and novel biomarkers

Classical biomarkers (e.g., ADA, CEA, CRP) continue to be widely utilized in the etiological differentiation of pleural effusions; however, they have limitations in terms of specificity, sensitivity, and early diagnostic capability. Consequently, research into next-generation biomarkers has gained momentum in recent years. These novel markers aim to detect disease at the molecular level earlier and, in some cases, provide prognostic information.

7.1. Osteopontin

Osteopontin is a secreted glycoprotein that facilitates tissue repair following injury or infection. It regulates cellular migration and stimulates intracellular signaling via its interaction with multiple cell surface receptors [59]. Additionally, it plays a significant role in modulating immune and inflammatory responses. Osteopontin is associated with cellular adhesion and tumor invasion. Studies have indicated that osteopontin levels may aid in distinguishing malignant pleural mesothelioma from benign pleural effusions [60]. This biomarker also shows potential as a prognostic indicator.

7.2. High-mobility group box 1 (HMGB1)

HMGB1 is a nuclear protein that binds DNA non-specifically and functions as a chromatin-binding factor. It plays roles in DNA repair, transcription, cell differentiation, extracellular signaling, and somatic recombination. HMGB1 is released during necrosis and actively secreted during inflammation. Elevated HMGB1 levels have been detected in both malignant and infectious pleural effusions [61].

7.3. IL-18, IL-36, and other cytokines

IL-18: IL-18 is involved in the regulation of both innate and adaptive immune responses and plays a significant role in autoimmune, inflammatory, and infectious diseases [62]. It contributes to the differentiation of naïve T cells into Th1 cells and stimulates IFN-γ production by T cells and natural killer (NK) cells. IL-18 enhances the pro-inflammatory response in tuberculosis and parapneumonic effusions [63, 64].

IL-36: Interleukin-36 (IL-36) is a newly recognized pro-inflammatory cytokine in the IL-1 family. IL-36 acts on keratinocytes, lymphocytes, monocytes/macrophages, and plasma cells. It has been implicated in the progression of malignancies, pneumonia, and tuberculosis. In complicated parapneumonic effusions, IL-36 levels are elevated in conjunction with other members of the IL-1 family [65].

8. The role of biomarkers in clinical decision-making

In the differential diagnosis of pleural effusions, classical approaches – clinical evaluation, imaging findings, and Light's criteria – often fall short. Therefore, the appropriate selection and use of biomarkers within structured diagnostic algorithms play a critical role in minimizing invasive procedures, enabling early diagnosis, and guiding treatment strategies.

8.1. Role of biomarkers in diagnostic algorithms

- Tuberculosis: The combination of ADA >40 IU/L, IFN-γ, and IL-27 can facilitate diagnosis without the need for a biopsy [66].

- Malignancy suspicion: In patients with CEA >5 ng/mL and positive mesothelin or fibulin-3, the necessity for thoracoscopy may be reduced.

- Parapneumonic effusions: High levels of CRP (>100 mg/L), PCT (>0.5 ng/mL), and elevated MIF increase the likelihood of a complicated effusion.

8.2. Reducing the need for invasive procedures

High-specificity biomarkers allow for the reduction of invasive procedures, such as biopsy or thoracoscopy, particularly in cases of suspected malignancy or tuberculosis.

8.3. Biomarkers in guiding treatment strategies

- Antibiotic decisions: Elevated PCT levels may predict empyema development and support early drainage.

- Tuberculosis therapy: Early treatment can be initiated in patients with high ADA and IFN-γ.

- Oncological management: Persistently elevated mesothelin levels may indicate disease progression and the need for chemotherapy adjustments.

8.4. Monitoring and prognostic evaluation

Recent studies highlight the prognostic value of sST2 levels in pleural fluid, particularly in effusions related to heart failure and pulmonary hypertension.

8.5. Invasive approaches when necessary

When diagnostic uncertainty persists, or when there is a strong suspicion of malignancy, tuberculosis, or complicated infections, invasive procedures such as thoracoscopy should be considered. Thoracoscopy remains the gold standard for histologic confirmation in malignant pleural diseases.

9. Conclusion and future perspectives

Etiologic diagnosis of pleural effusion remains one of the most complex and multifactorial challenges in clinical practice. Recent advances in biomarker discovery have not only improved diagnostic accuracy but also enhanced prognostic assessment, reduced the need for invasive procedures, and informed treatment decisions.

This chapter has comprehensively reviewed the diagnostic and prognostic roles of classical and emerging pleural biomarkers – including ADA, CEA, mesothelin, fibulin-3, IFN-γ, PCT, sST2, and HMGB1 – across various etiologies such as parapneumonic, tuberculous, malignant, transudative, and autoimmune effusions.

Biomarker-based diagnostic algorithms and clinical decision-support strategies have also been presented. Liquid biopsy technologies, particularly in malignancy, are proving promising for providing detailed insights into pathological processes through the analysis of extracellular vesicles (exosomes), microRNAs, and circulating tumor DNA (ctDNA).

The integration of multiparametric biomarker panels may facilitate the development of more sensitive and accurate etiological classification systems for pleural fluid in the near future.

Artificial intelligence-assisted decision systems may expedite clinical decisions by automatically analyzing complex biomarker data.

Well-designed, prospective, multicenter, biomarker-focused clinical trials will be essential for integrating these biomarkers into standard diagnostic protocols.

In conclusion, pleural biomarkers are expected to become an increasingly integral component of future clinical practice, forming the foundation for personalized diagnostics and

List of abbreviations

MPE	Malignant pleural effusion
ADA	Adenosine deaminase
CRP	C-Reactive protein
CEA	Carcinoembryonic antigen
IL	Interleukin
NSE	Neuron-specific enolase
VEGF	Vascular endothelial growth factor
AFP	Alpha-fetoprotein
SCC	Squamous cell carcinoma antigen
ATT	Anti-tuberculosis therapy
TPE	Tuberculous pleural effusion
IFN-γ	Interferon-gamma
ESAT-6	Early secretory antigen-6
IGRA	Interferon-gamma release assays
PCT	Procalcitonin
PPPE	Parapneumonic pleural effusions
NT-proBNP	N-terminal Pro-B-type natriuretic peptide
BNP	Brain natriuretic peptide
Soluble ST2	Suppression of the tumorigenesis-2 receptor
TrPE	Transudative pleural effusion
MIF	Macrophage migration inhibitory factor
ANA	Antinuclear antibody
Anti-dsDNA	Anti-double stranded DNA
RF	Rheumatoid factor
MIP-3α	Macrophage inflammatory Protein 3 alpha
HMGB1	High-mobility group box 1
NK	Natural killer
ctDNA	Circulating tumor DNA

Conflict of interest

The authors declare no conflicts of interest.

Author details

Fatma Selen Ala Çitlak
Çarşamba State Hospital, Çarşamba/SAMSUN, Türkiye

*Address all correspondence to: selennala@gmail.com

References

[1] Zhang M, Li D, Zd H, YL H. The diagnostic utility of pleural markers for tuberculosis pleural effusion. Annals of Translational Medicine. 2020;**8**(9):607

[2] Shi H-Z, Liang Q-L, Jiang J, Qin X-J, YANG H-B. Diagnostic value of carcinoembryonic antigen in malignant pleural effusion: A meta-analysis. Respirology. 2008;**13**(4):518–527

[3] Porcel JM.Pleural fluid biomarkers: Beyond the Light criteria. Clinics in Chest Medicine. 2013;**34**(1):27–37

[4] Görgün D, Seçik F, Midilli K, Akkaya V, Yıldız P. Diagnostic and prognostic significance of survivin levels in malignant pleural effusion. Respiratory Medicine. 2013;**107** (8):1260–1265

[5] Cincin A, Abul Y, Ozben B, Tanrikulu A, Topaloglu N, Ozgul G, et al. Pleural fluid amino-terminal brain natriuretic peptide in patients with pleural effusions. Respiratory Care. 2013;**58**:313–319

[6] Davies HE, Sadler RS, Bielsa S, Maskell NA, Rahman NM, Davies RJ, et al. Clinical impact and reliability of pleural fluid mesothelin in undiagnosed pleural effusions. American Journal of Respiratory and Critical Care Medicine. 2009;**180**:437–444

[7] Guo L, Zhang Q, Lv C, Ma X, Song X, Huang J, et al.. A novel biomarker for pleural effusion diagnosis: Interleukin-36 γ in pleural fluid. Journal of Clinical Laboratory Analysis. 2023;**37**(1)

[8] Porcel JM, Galindo C, Esquerda A, Trujillano J, Ruiz-González A, Falguera M, et al. Pleural fluid interleukin-8 and C-reactive protein for discriminating complicated non-purulent from uncomplicated parapneumonic effusions. Respirology. 2008;**13**:58–62

[9] Scherpereel A, Grigoriu B, Conti M, Gey T, Grégoire M, Copin MC, et al. Soluble mesothelin-related peptides in the diagnosis of malignant pleural mesothelioma. American Journal of Respiratory and Critical Care Medicine. 2006;**173**:1155–1160

[10] San José ME, Valdes L, Gonzalez-Barcala FJ, Vizcaino L, Garrido M, Sanmartin A, et al. Diagnostic value of proinflammatory interleukins in parapneumonic effusions. American Journal of Clinical Pathology. 2010;**133**:884–891

[11] Romero-Candeira S, Fernández C, Martín C, Sánchez-Paya J, Hernández L. Influence of diuretics on the concentration of proteins and other components of pleural transudates in patients with heart failure. American Journal of Medicine. 2001;**110**(9):681–686

[12] Ren R, Yin P, Zhang Y, Zhou J, Zhou Y, Xu R, et al. Diagnostic value of fibulin-3 for malignant pleural mesothelioma: A systematic review and meta-analysis. Oncotarget. 2016;7:84851–84859

[13] Liang QL, Shi HZ, Qin XJ, Liang XD, Jiang J, Yang HB. Diagnostic accuracy of tumour markers for malignant pleural effusion: A meta-analysis. Thorax. 2008;**63**(1):35–41

[14] Alataş F, Alataş O, Metintaş M, Colak O, Harmanci E, Demir S. Diagnostic value of CEA, CA 15-3, CA

19-9, CYFRA 21-1, NSE and TSA assay in pleural effusions. Lung Cancer. 2001;**31**(1):9–16

[15] Zhang Y, Wang J, Liang B, Wu H, Chen Y. Diagnosis of malignant pleural effusion with combinations of multiple tumor markers: A comparison study of five machine learning models. International Journal of Biological Markers. 2023;**38**(2):139–146

[16] Han CH, Choi JE, Chung JH. Clinical utility of pleural fluid NT-pro brain natriuretic peptide (NT-proBNP) in patients with pleural effusions. Internal Medicine. 2008;**47**(19):1669–1674

[17] Schuetz P, Mueller B.To escalate or to de-escalte–that is the question. Critical Care Medicine. 2011;**39**(11):2590

[18] Grove CS, Lee YC. Vascular endothelial growth factor: The key mediator in pleural effusion formation. Current Opinion in Pulmonary Medicine. 2002;**8**(4):294–301

[19] Fiorelli A, Vicidomini G, Di Domenico M, Napolitano F, Messina G, Morgillo F, et al. Vascular endothelial growth factor in pleural fluid for differential diagnosis of benign and malignant origin and its clinical applications. Interactive Cardiovascular and Thoracic Surgery. 2011;**12**:420–424

[20] Denhardt DT, Noda M. Osteopontin expression and function: Role in bone remodeling. Journal of Cellular Biochemistry. 1998;**72**(S30-31):92–102

[21] Elgwairi E, Abdalla A, Elkheshen A, Elharabi Z, Nugent K. Pleural Effusions in Patients With Congestive Heart Failure: Frequency, Pathogenesis, Diagnosis, and Implications. Cardiology in Review. 2024;**32**(2):91–96

[22] Kim SJ, Hwang SO, Kim YW, Lee JH, Cha KC. Procalcitonin as a diagnostic marker for sepsis/septic shock in the emergency department; a study based on Sepsis-3 definition. American Journal of Emergency Medicine. 2019;**37**(2):272–276

[23] Pascual-Figal DA, Ordoñez-Llanos J, Tornel PL, Vázquez R, Puig T, Valdés M, et al. Soluble ST2 for predicting sudden cardiac death in patients with chronic heart failure and left ventricular systolic dysfunction. Journal of the American College of Cardiology. 2009;**54**:2174–2179

[24] Kiropoulos TS, Kostikas K, Oikonomidi S, Tsilioni I, Nikoulis D, Germenis A, et al. Acute phase markers for the differentiation of infectious and malignant pleural effusions. Respiratory Medicine. 2007;**101**:910–918

[25] Chen Z, Gaudino G, Pass HI, Carbone M, Yang H. Diagnostic and prognostic biomarkers for malignant mesothelioma: An update. Translational Lung Cancer Research. 2017;**6**(3):259–269

[26] Bielsa S, Porcel JM, Castellote J, Mas E, Esquerda A, Light RW. Solving the Light's criteria misclassification rate of cardiac and hepatic transudates. Respirology. 2012;**17**(4):721–726

[27] Song CH, Lee JS, Nam HH, Kim JM, Suhr JW, Jung SS, et al. IL-18 production in human pulmonary and pleural tuberculosis. Scandinavian Journal of Immunology. 2002;**56**:611–618

[28] Pass HI, Levin SM, Harbut MR, Melamed J, Chiriboga L, Donington J, et al. Fibulin-3 as a blood and effusion

biomarker for pleural mesothelioma. New England Journal of Medicine. 2012;**367**:1417–1427

[29] Villena Garrido V, Cases Viedma E, Fernández Villar A, de Pablo Gafas A, Pérez Rodríguez E, Porcel Pérez JM, et al. Recommendations of diagnosis and treatment of pleural effusion. Archivos de Bronconeumología. 2014;**50**:235–249

[30] O'Dwyer MJ, Mankan AK, White M, Lawless MW, Stordeur P, O'Connell B, et al. The human response to infection is associated with distinct patterns of interleukin 23 and interleukin 27 expression. Intensive Care Medicine. 2008;**34**:683–691

[31] Zhang M, Yan L, Lippi G, Hu Z-D. Pleural biomarkers in diagnostics of malignant pleural effusion: A narrative review. Translational Lung Cancer Research. 2021;**10**(3):1557–1570

[32] San José ME, Valdés L, Vizcaíno LH, Mora T, Pose A, Soneira E, et al. Procalcitonin, C-reactive protein, and cell counts in the diagnosis of parapneumonic pleural effusions. Journal of Investigative Medicine. 2010;**58**:971–976

[33] Wu YB, Ye ZJ, Qin SM, Wu C, Chen YQ, Shi HZ. Combined detections of interleukin 27, interferon-γ, and adenosine deaminase in pleural effusion for diagnosis of tuberculous pleurisy. Chinese Medical Journal (English). 2013;**126**(17):3215–3221

[34] Yang CY, Kuo YH, Chen M, Wang CL, Shih LJ, Liu YC, et al. Pleural cytokines MIF and MIP-3α as novel biomarkers for complicated parapneumonic effusions and empyema. Scientific Reports. 2021;**11**:1763

[35] Volarić D, Flego V, Žauhar G, Bulat-Kardum L. Diagnostic value of tumour markers in pleural effusions. Biochemia Medica (Zagreb). 2018;**28** (1):010706

[36] Muley T, Dienemann H, Herth FJ, Thomas M, Meister M, Schneider J. Combination of mesothelin and CEA significantly improves the differentiation between malignant pleural mesothelioma, benign asbestos disease, and lung cancer. Journal of Thoracic Oncology. 2013;**8**(7):947–951

[37] Aggarwal AN, Agarwal R, Dhooria S, Prasad KT, Sehgal IS, Muthu V. Comparative accuracy of pleural fluid unstimulated interferon-gamma and adenosine deaminase for diagnosing pleural tuberculosis: A systematic review and meta-analysis. PLoS One. 2021;**16**(6)

[38] Shaw JA, Diacon AH, Koegelenberg CFN. Tuberculous pleural effusion. Respirology. 2019;**24**(10):962–971

[39] Kurt M, Akdeniz M, Kavukcu E. Assessment of Comorbidity and Use of Prescription and Nonprescription Drugs in Patients Above 65 Years Attending Family Medicine Outpatient Clinics. Gerontology and Geriatric Medicine. 2019;**5**:2333721419874274

[40] Kotsiou OS, Jagirdar RM, Papazoglou ED, Hatzoglou C, Gourgoulianis KI, Zarogiannis SG. Pleural effusion IL-33/sST2 levels and effects of low and high IL-33/sST2 levels on human mesothelial cell adhesion and migration. Inflammation. 2019;**42** (6):2072–2085

[41] Sugawara I, Yamada H, Kaneko H, Mizuno S, Takeda K, Akira S. Role of interleukin-18 (IL-18) in mycobacterial

infection in IL-18-gene-disrupted mice. Infection and Immunity. 1999;**67** (5):2585–2589

[42] Song X, Guo L, Zhang Q, Chen W, Fan W, Lv C, et al. The diagnostic value of interleukin-36 cytokines in Pleural Effusions of varying etiologies. Clinica Chimica Acta. 2023;**549**:117533

[43] Dheda K, Van-Zyl Smit RN, Sechi LA, Badri M, Meldau R, Symons G, et al.. Clinical diagnostic utility of IP-10 and LAM antigen levels for the diagnosis of tuberculous pleural effusions in a high burden setting. PLOS ONE. 2009;**4**(3)

[44] Yeh JH, Huang CT, Liu CH, Ruan SY, Tsai YJ, Chien YC, et al.. Cautious application of pleural N-terminal pro-B-type natriuretic peptide in diagnosis of congestive heart failure pleural effusions among critically ill patients. PLoS One. 2014;**9**(12)

[45] Wu KM, Chang WK, Chen CH, Kou YR. Expression of IL-1β, HMGB1, HO-1, and LDH in malignant and non-malignant pleural effusions. Respiratory Physiology & Neurobiology. 2020;**272**:103330

[46] He C, Wang B, Li D, Xu H, Yongchun S. Performance of procalcitonin in diagnosing parapneumonic pleural effusions: A clinical study and meta-analysis. Medicine. 2017;96:e7829

[47] Creaney J, Dick IM, Meniawy TM, Leong SL, Leon JS, Demelker Y, et al. Comparison of fibulin-3 and mesothelin as markers in malignant mesothelioma. Thorax. 2014;**69**:895–902

[48] Chen DY, Huang YH, Chen YM, Chen JJW, Yang TY, Chang GC, et al.. ANA positivity and complement level in pleural fluid are potential diagnostic markers in discriminating lupus pleuritis from pleural effusion of other aetiologies. Lupus Science & Medicine. 2021;**8**(1)

[49] Valdés L, San José E, Alvarez D, Valle JM.Adenosine Deaminase (ADA) isoenzyme analysis in pleural effusions: Diagnostic role, and relevance to the origin of increased ADA in Tuberculous pleurisy. European Respiratory Journal. 1996;**9**(4):747–751

[50] Pang CS, Shen YC, Tian PW, Zhu J, Feng M, Wan C, et al. Accuracy of the interferon-gamma release assay for the Diagnosis of Tuberculous pleurisy: An Updated Meta-Analysis. PeerJournal. 2015;**3**:e951

[51] Jiang J, Shi HZ, Liang QL, SM Q, XJ Q. Diagnostic value of Interferon-Gamma in tuberculous pleurisy: A meta analysis. Chest. 2007;**131**(4):1133–1141

[52] Hirayama N, Tabata C, Tabata R, Maeda R, Yasumitsu A, Yamada S, et al. Pleural effusion VEGF levels as a prognostic factor of malignant pleural mesothelioma. Respiratory Medicine. 2011;**105**:137–142

[53] Tomita M, Shimizu T, Matsuzaki Y, Hara M, Ayabe T, Onitsuka T. Prognostic Significance of carcinoembryonic antigen level in pleural lavage fluid for patients with lung Adenocarcinoma. The Annals of Thoracic Surgery. 2005;**80** (1):276–281

[54] Porcel JM, Vives M, Cao G, Esquerda A, Rubio M, Rivas MC. Measurement of pro-brain natriuretic peptide in pleural fluid for the diagnosis of pleural effusions due to heart failure. American Journal of Medicine. 2004;**116**(6):417–420

[55] Hollevoet K, Nackaerts K, Gosselin R, De Wever W, Bosquée L, De Vuyst P, et al. Soluble mesothelin, megakaryocyte potentiating factor, and osteopontin as markers of patient response and outcome in mesothelioma. Journal of Thoracic Oncology. 2011;**6**:1930–1937

[56] Li H, Luo YF, Blackwell TS, Xie CM. Meta-analysis and systematic review of procalcitonin-guided therapy in respiratory tract infections. Antimicrobial Agents and Chemotherapy. 2011;**55**(12):5900–5906

[57] mA S, Valeh T, Ehteram H, Haddad Kashani H, Ghazi Zahedi M. Diagnostic Value of Neuron-Specific Enolase (NSE) and Cancer Antigen 15-3 (CA 15-3) in the Diagnosis of Pleural Effusions. Asian Pacific Journal of Cancer Prevention. 2017;**18**(1):257–261

[58] Liang QL, Shi HZ, Wang K, Qin SM, Qin XJ. Diagnostic accuracy of adenosine deaminase in tuberculous pleurisy: A meta-analysis. Respiratory Medicine. 2008;**102**(5):744–754

[59] Roy B, Shak HJ, Lee YCG. Pleural fluid investigations for pleural infections. Journal of Laboratory and Precision Medicine. 2021;**6**

[60] Biet F, Locht C, Kremer L. Immunoregulatory functions of interleukin 18 and its role in defense against bacterial pathogens. Journal of Molecular Medicine (Berlin). 2002;**80**(3):147–162

[61] Görgün D, Seçik F, Midilli K, Akkaya V, Yıldız P.Diagnostic and prognostic significance of survivin levels in malignant pleural effusion. Respiratory Medicine. 2013;**107**(8):1260–1265

[62] Jeon D. Tuberculous pleurisy: An update. Tuberculosis and Respiratory Diseases (Seoul). 2014;**76**(4):153–159

[63] Yang Q, Cha SN, Niu Y, Wen JX, Yan L, Hai L, et al. Diagnostic Utility of Pleural C-Reactive Protein and Procalcitonin for Parapneumonic Pleural Effusion: A Head-to-Head Comparison Study. Infection and Drug Resistance. 2025;**18**:919–927

[64] Psallidas I, Kalomenidis I, Porcel JM, Robinson BW, Stathopoulos GT. Malignant pleural effusion: From bench to bedside. European Respiratory Review. 2016;**25**(140):189–198

[65] Bradshaw M, Mansfield A, Peikert T. The role of vascular endothelial growth factor in the pathogenesis, diagnosis and treatment of malignant pleural effusion. Current Oncology Reports. 2013;**15**(3):207–216

[66] He T, Oh S. Diagnostic approach to pleural effusions. AME Medical Journal. 2018;**3**

Section 4

Surgical Management of Pleural Disease

Chapter 8

Pleural Decortication in the Era of Minimally Invasive Thoracic Surgery: The Role of VATS

Güntuğ Batıhan

Abstract

Pleural decortication is a fundamental operation for restoring lung expansion in organized pleural disease. Over the last two decades, video-assisted thoracoscopic surgery (VATS) has evolved from a drainage-and-debridement tool to a definitive decortication approach for selected patients with organized empyema, retained hemothorax, and trapped lung from chronic pleuritis or hemothorax. Compared with open thoracotomy, VATS decortication is associated with less postoperative pain, shorter length of stay, and faster recovery, while maintaining comparable success rates when complete parietal and visceral pleural peel removal can be achieved. Patient selection, stage-based timing, and meticulous subpleural plane dissection are the cornerstones of efficacy. This chapter outlines indications, work-up, anesthesia and positioning, step-by-step VATS technique (multiport and uniportal), decision thresholds for conversion, management of complex scenarios (tuberculous and fungal empyema, postlobectomy space, bronchopleural fistula, retained hemothorax, pediatric cases), postoperative care (including digital drain strategies), complication avoidance and management (persistent air leak, bleeding, reexpansion pulmonary edema), and expected outcomes. We also summarize the current evidence base and practical algorithms to guide adoption in low- and high-volume centers, and highlight future directions, including robotic assistance, image-guided dissection, and data-driven drain management.

Keywords: video-assisted thoracoscopic surgery (VATS), pleural decortication, empyema, trapped lung, retained hemothorax, minimally invasive thoracic surgery, bronchopleural fistula

1. Introduction

Pleural diseases that restrict lung excursion – most classically chronic empyema and organized hemothorax – can progress to a dense visceral and parietal peel that mechanically traps the lung. The resulting loss of pleural apposition perpetuates infection, impairs gas exchange, and creates a residual space prone to ongoing sepsis and prolonged hospitalization. When antibiotics, image-guided drainage, and intrapleural therapies do not restore full expansion, surgical decortication becomes the definitive treatment to reexpand the lung, obliterate the cavity, and eradicate infection [1–4].

1.1 Why decortication matters

The fibrous peel reduces lung compliance, elevates pleural pressures, and limits diaphragmatic excursion. Removing this rind restores the subpleural sliding plane, permits effective ventilation of previously atelectatic segments, and facilitates early mobilization and secretion clearance. Timely surgery can shorten the course of antibiotics, reduce drain dependency, and prevent chronic fibrothorax. In malignant or noninfective trapped lung, carefully selected decortication can also palliate dyspnea and improve quality of life.

1.2 Evolution toward minimally invasive surgery

Historically, thoracotomy was the standard approach for organized empyema and fibrothorax. Over the past two decades, video-assisted thoracoscopic surgery (VATS) has transitioned from a drainage/debridement tool to a platform capable of complete parietal and visceral decortication in selected patients. Endoscopic magnification aids in the identification of the subpleural plane, while reduced chest wall trauma translates into less pain, lower wound morbidity, shorter length of stay, and faster functional recovery. In contemporary series, VATS achieves comparable clearance and reexpansion rates to open surgery when the correct plane can be developed, with conversion used judiciously as a safety strategy rather than a failure [5, 6].

1.3 Where VATS fits in the treatment pathway

Modern care is algorithmic. Early phases of pleural infection or hemothorax often respond to image-guided tube thoracostomy and intrapleural enzymes. Progression to the organizing phase, persistent loculation with nonexpanding lung, or failure of medical therapy are clear triggers for operative intervention. VATS is the preferred first-line surgical approach in most cases of organized disease without extensive calcification, complex chest wall defects, or unstable physiology. Patient selection hinges on imaging (peel thickness, calcification, fissural involvement), etiology (tuberculous/fungal vs. bacterial), duration of symptoms, and the anticipated ability to develop a safe subpleural plane [7–9].

1.4 Safety, conversion, and outcomes

The primary goals are the complete evacuation of infected material, the removal of parietal and visceral rind sufficient to allow full reexpansion, and meticulous hemostasis. Conversion to thoracotomy should occur early when the plane is unsafe, bleeding is uncontrolled, or expansion remains inadequate – prioritizing patient safety over approach fidelity. With this philosophy, VATS decortication in appropriately selected patients yields high success rates, low wound morbidity, and rapid convalescence. Predictors of technical difficulty include long symptom duration, tuberculous etiology, severe malnutrition, and calcified rind.

1.5 Scope of this chapter

This chapter offers a practical, surgeon-centered roadmap for VATS decortication. We outline indications and timing, preoperative assessment, anesthesia and positioning, instruments, multiport and uniportal techniques, conversion thresholds, and management of complex scenarios (tuberculous disease, retained hemothorax, bronchopleural fistula (BPF), postresection spaces, pediatric cases, and malignant trapped lung). We then detail postoperative pathways – including digital drain strategies – and strategies for complication avoidance and management. Finally, we summarize the evidence base, discuss the learning curve and resource considerations for low- and high-volume centers, and highlight future directions such as robotic assistance and image-guided dissection.

2. Pathophysiology and staging of pleural organization

Parapneumonic effusions and hemothorax evolve along a biological continuum driven by inflammation, disordered coagulation–fibrinolysis, and fibroblast ingrowth. Clinically, the process typically begins with an exudative phase in which increased pleural permeability produces a sterile, protein-rich effusion. At this stage, ultrasound often shows anechoic or only minimally complex fluid, and computed tomography (CT) may be unremarkable apart from the effusion; with timely tube thoracostomy, many patients improve without further intervention. Progression to the fibrinopurulent phase is marked by bacterial invasion and neutrophil activation, with rises in pro-inflammatory cytokines (such as IL-6 and TNF-α) and plasminogen activator inhibitor-1, tipping the balance toward fibrin deposition and failure of fibrinolysis. Septations and loculations form, pleural fluid pH and glucose fall, and LDH increases. Ultrasound at this point reveals fibrous strands and echogenic debris, while CT commonly demonstrates the split-pleura sign and early pleural thickening. In the organizing phase, fibroblasts and myofibroblasts migrate along the fibrin scaffold and deposit collagen, creating a dense visceral and parietal rind. Neovascularization renders the pleura hypervascular. The visceral peel restricts alveolar expansion and stiffens the lung, producing the physiology of a trapped lung [10, 11].

The timing of these transitions is variable, but exudative changes are usually predominant over the first few days; fibrinopurulence emerges by days 3–7, and organization can appear after one to two weeks. This trajectory accelerates with virulent organisms, delayed drainage, diabetes, malnutrition, renal failure, or immunosuppression. Tuberculous and fungal pleuritis characteristically generate a thick, hypervascular, and sometimes calcified rind with dense fissural adhesions and pleural space calcification – features that predict longer operations, greater bleeding risk, and a higher likelihood of conversion. In retained hemothorax, polymerized fibrin within the clot provides an ideal scaffold for fibroblast ingrowth, and failure to evacuate the collection can culminate in fibrothorax [12–14].

Physiologically, it is helpful to distinguish lung entrapment from trapped lung. Lung entrapment reflects impaired expansion due to active pleural inflammation and often improves as inflammation resolves. Trapped lung denotes a chronic fibrotic visceral peel that mechanically prevents reexpansion; pleural manometry in these cases shows high elastance with a steep pressure–volume curve and failure of pressure equilibration during drainage. This distinction informs surgical timing and frames postoperative expectations. The overall approach and treatment strategy for empyema are summarized in the diagram shown in **Figure 1**.

Imaging and bedside physiology provide complementary staging. Ultrasound differentiates free from complex-septated effusions, maps loculations for port planning, and the loss of pleural glide may suggest a visceral rind. CT depicts pleural thickening and enhancement, the split-pleura sign, loculations, patterns of atelectasis, diaphragmatic involvement, and calcification, thereby helping anticipate whether a thoracoscopic plane can be developed. Where available, pleural manometry demonstrating elevated elastance (for example, >14–20 cmH_2O/L) supports a nonexpandable lung physiology. Surgically, the target is the relatively avascular subpleural (submesothelial) areolar plane superficial to the visceral pleura. Development of this plane allows the visceral rind to be shelled out with traction–counter-traction while preserving alveolar integrity. When inflammation obliterates or calcifies this interface – particularly across fissures or over the diaphragm – safe progress may require staged dissection, limited "window" decortications, or early conversion to thoracotomy to prevent lung tears and uncontrolled bleeding [15–17].

Operationally, early exudative disease is usually managed with image-guided drainage and antibiotics, whereas fibrinopurulent disease warrants drainage with adjunctive intrapleural tPA/DNase or early VATS in the setting of multiloculation or nonexpansion. In the organizing phase, VATS decortication is feasible for many patients but carries a higher conversion risk; a primary open approach should be considered when there is extensive calcification, tuberculous or fungal etiology with obliterated planes, or hemodynamic fragility. A precise grasp of this biology–imaging–physiology triad guides case selection, timing, port strategy, and the threshold for conversion in VATS decortication.

3. Preoperative evaluation and patient selection

Preoperative evaluation aims to define the extent of pleural organization, anticipate the feasibility of a safe subpleural plane, and optimize the patient for single-lung anesthesia. Contrast-enhanced chest CT is the workhorse to delineate loculations, peel thickness and distribution, fissural and diaphragmatic involvement, lung-collapse patterns, and adhesions. Bedside thoracic ultrasound complements CT by mapping septations, identifying the most accessible pocket for entry, and informing port planning; absent pleural glide and a calcified rind on imaging both predict technical difficulty.

Microbiological assessment should include pleural fluid Gram stain and culture, with acid-fast bacilli testing when tuberculosis is suspected; antimicrobial therapy is then tailored to the results and local epidemiology. Pulmonary evaluation with spirometry (where feasible) helps set expectations and guides perioperative rehabilitation; early mobilization and preoperative incentive spirometry are encouraged to enhance postoperative recovery [18, 19].

Risk stratification focuses on correctable factors – nutritional status (e.g., serum albumin), anemia, glycemic control, and perioperative anticoagulation management – alongside the assessment of comorbidities that might impair tolerance of single-lung ventilation. In addition, formal risk assessment tools such as the RAPID score (Renal, Age, Purulence, Infection source, and Dietary factors) and the Charlson Comorbidity Index (CCI) can help predict short- and long-term outcomes

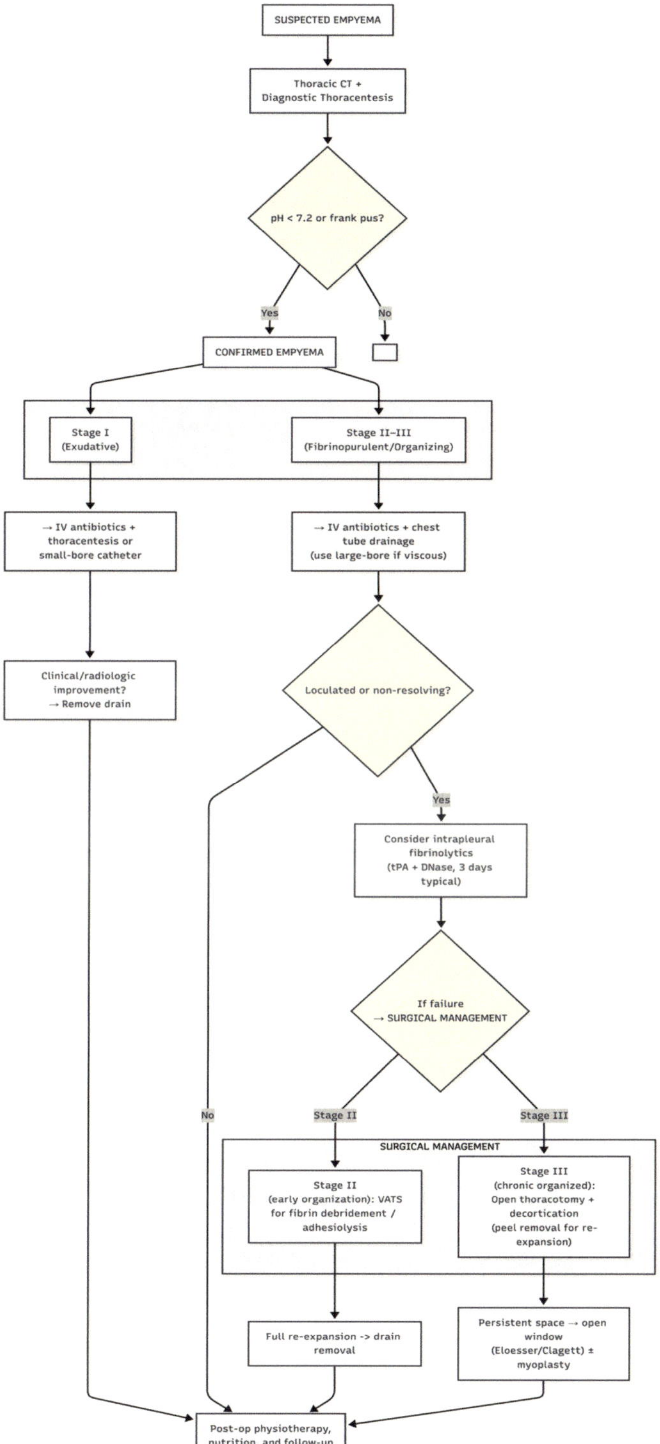

Figure 1.
Stage-Based Management Algorithm for Pleural Empyema.

in pleural infection and guide patient selection for surgery. Patients with high RAPID scores (≥5) are at increased risk of mortality and may benefit from early multidisciplinary input, while a higher CCI reflects systemic vulnerability and supports preoperative optimization rather than immediate intervention [20, 21]. Integrating these structured scores with imaging and physiologic findings allows for a more objective, individualized surgical decision-making process. The anesthesia plan should specify the method for lung isolation (double-lumen endotracheal tube or bronchial blocker) and incorporate regional analgesia (erector spinae plane or paravertebral block) within a multimodal strategy.

Patients in whom single-lung ventilation cannot be achieved, those with severe pleural calcification that obliterates the subpleural plane, hemodynamic instability, uncontrolled sepsis, or complex chest wall defects requiring open reconstruction are poor candidates for a primary thoracoscopic approach. In such settings, staged optimization or an upfront open strategy may be safer.

4. Anesthesia, positioning, and equipment

For VATS decortication, the patient is placed in full lateral decubitus with the table flexed to widen the intercostal spaces, and all pressure points are carefully padded. In selected cases with bilateral disease, sequential or dual-position strategies may be used to allow staged access. Lung isolation is achieved as planned preoperatively, and protective single-lung ventilation is maintained with low tidal volumes and appropriate PEEP, with periodic recruitment of the dependent lung; permissive hypercapnia is acceptable in hemodynamically stable patients.

Analgesia follows a multimodal approach. A regional block – typically an erector spinae plane or paravertebral block – is combined with local intercostal infiltration at port sites and nonopioid systemic agents. High-dose opioids are avoided where possible to facilitate early mobilization and effective physiotherapy.

Essential equipment includes a 30° thoracoscope; long, narrow periosteal elevators; peanut dissectors; ring forceps; suction-dissectors; bipolar or ultrasonic energy devices; and endoscopic cotton/tampon swabs. Long graspers aid traction on the peel during subpleural dissection. Where available, a digital chest-drain device is preferred to guide postoperative suction and removal using objective air-leak trends.

5. Operative technique – VATS decortication

The operative objective is threefold: eradicate infected/organized material, restore full lung reexpansion by removing parietal and visceral rind in the correct subpleural plane, and exit the chest with secure hemostasis and a drain strategy that promotes recovery rather than complications. The technique should be reproducible, ergonomic, and explicitly safety-first – conversion is a tool, not a failure.

5.1 Port strategy

Multiport (three-port) VATS: the camera is placed in the 7th–8th intercostal space (ICS) at the mid-axillary line. Working ports are created in the 4th–5th ICS anterior-axillary line and the 7th–8th ICS posterior-axillary line, then fine-tuned to preoperative CT/ultrasound mapping of dominant loculations and the intended trajectory to the diaphragm and posterior gutter. Port geometry should permit relaxed triangulation to the fissures and hilum, with instrument shafts parallel rather than crossing.

Uniportal VATS: A 3–4 cm utility incision in the 4th–5th ICS (anterior-axillary line) accommodates a 30° thoracoscope (kept superior) and long, curved instruments (working inferiorly) to recreate triangulation (**Figure 2**). A wound protector preserves soft tissues and facilitates rapid instrument exchange. If exposure is inadequate or the plane is hostile, adding an accessory port early is prudent. An intraoperative view showing the operating table setup, port placement, and the surgeon's position is presented in **Figures 3a** and **3b**.

5.2 Entry and initial survey

Pleural entry is made through the safest pocket, guided by ultrasound as needed. After controlled aspiration and sampling for microbiology and cytology, blunt entry (finger or blunt trocar) minimizes parenchymal injury. The first goal is to convert multiple locules into a single working cavity by opening septations close to the chest wall (**Figure 4a–b**). Conduct a systematic survey – diaphragm, posterior gutter, fissures, hilum, mediastinum – identifying the phrenic nerve and intercostal bundles and planning the sequence of decortication. Warm irrigation improves visibility and maintains normothermia.

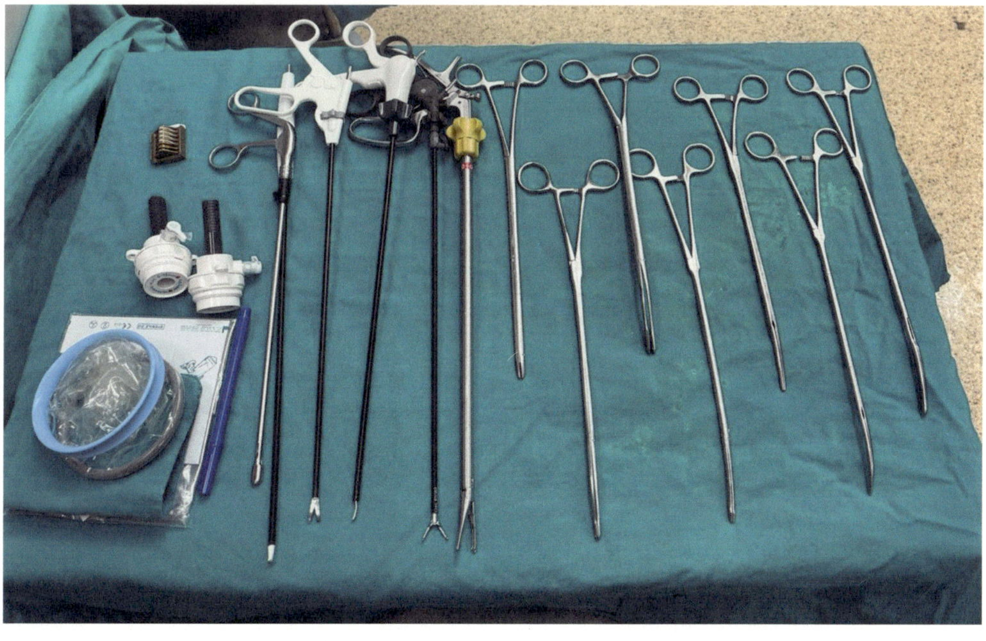

Figure 2.
Surgical Instrument Configuration for VATS Decortication.

5.3 Identifying the subpleural plane

Dissection begins over an atelectatic lobe where the rind is thickest and the plane easiest to demonstrate. Elevate the parietal peel gently with ring forceps and develop a cleavage plane superficial to the visceral pleura using a peanut or suction dissector held flat against the lung (**Figure 5a–b**). Short sweeping motions with steady traction–counter-traction advance the plane; small "peel windows" limit shear and

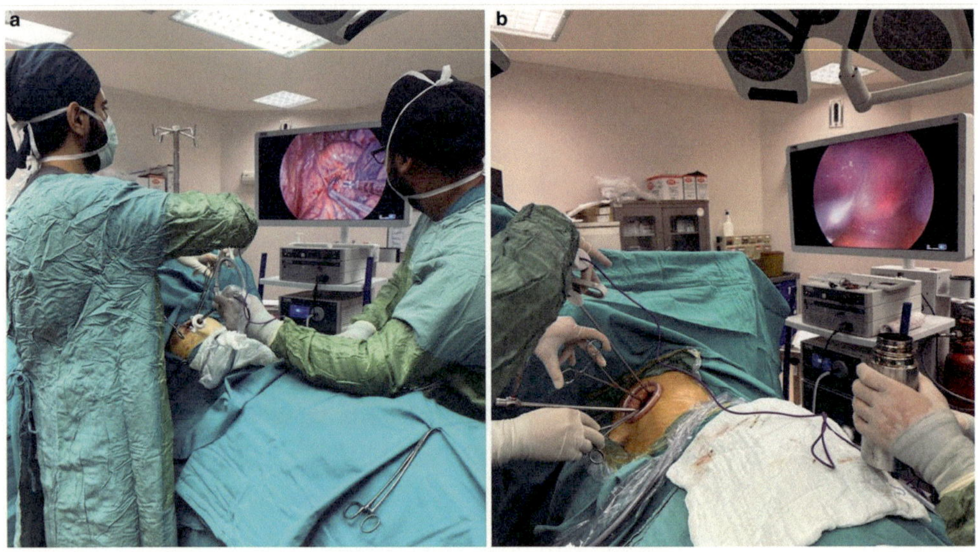

Figure 3.
Intraoperative Setup of Uniportal VATS: External Operative View.

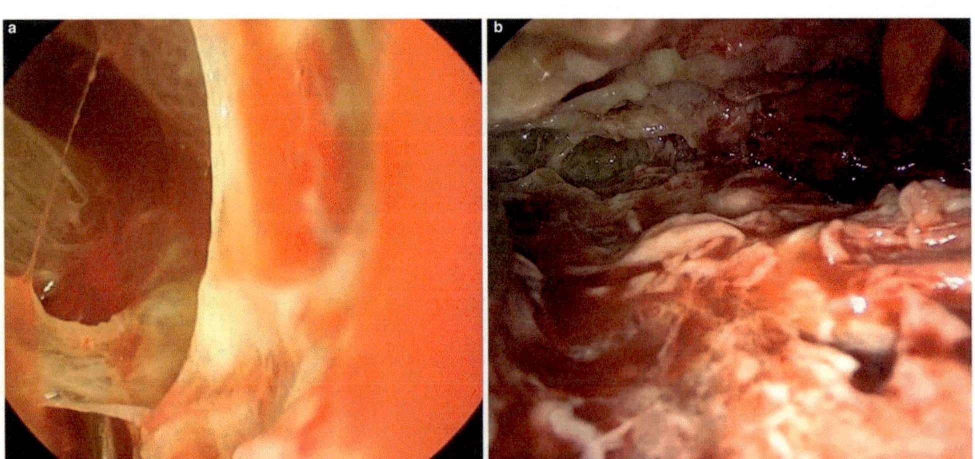

Figure 4.
Sequential Thoracoscopic Findings During VATS Decortication.

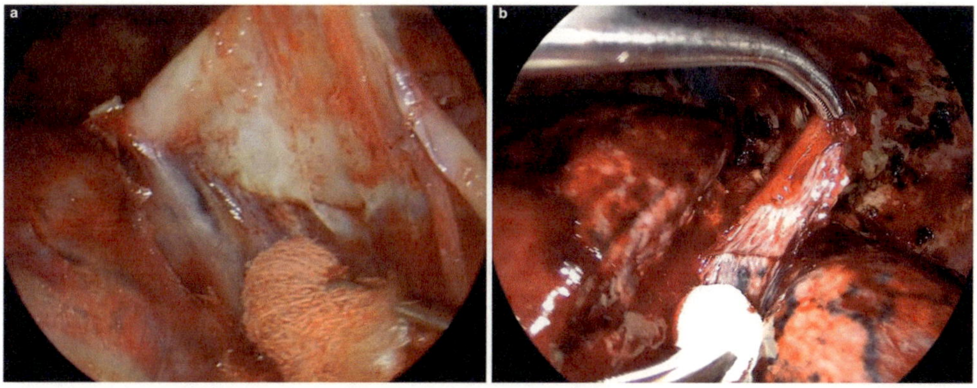

Figure 5.
Blunt Dissection Method for Visceral Decortication in VATS.

reduce lung tears (**Figure 6a–b**). Avoid using energy on the visceral surface; favor blunt and cold dissection. Intermittent reinflation confirms the adequacy of release and reveals areas where the plane is lost (brisk oozing from the lung surface or resistance to expansion).

5.4 Systematic decortication

Parietal component: begin with circumscribed removal of the parietal rind to create operating space, proceeding along the costal, diaphragmatic, and mediastinal pleura. Preserve the phrenic nerve on the pericardium, and avoid stripping directly over intercostal neurovascular bundles. On the diaphragm, gentle traction with peanut dissection minimizes muscle fiber bleeding.

Visceral component: shell the visceral rind from the hilum to the periphery in a segmental fashion, freeing the fissures last. Use narrow “trapdoor” windows rather than broad flaps when the plane is tenuous. Keep the lung moist; avoid desiccation, which obscures the plane and promotes air leaks. Near the hilum, respect bronchovascular structures; if a small parenchymal tear occurs, repair it with fine absorbable sutures on low insufflation and confirm with underwater testing.

Fissures and diaphragm: fissural bridges are divided with fine scissors in the established plane, keeping a wide berth from segmental vessels. Over the diaphragmatic dome, progress is made in short trenches directed toward the costophrenic recess, periodically reinflating to judge expansion and hemostasis.

5.5 Adjuncts

Warm irrigation clears debris and reduces tissue fragility. Hemostasis relies on bipolar/soft-coag with judicious topical agents (e.g., collagen or cellulose matrices) on oozing parietal beds; avoid thermal energy on visceral pleura. After decortication, perform a saline submersion test with incremental inflation to localize air leaks; manage with fine sutures, targeted sealant, or buttressing as indicated (**Figure 7a–b**). Send the rind for histopathology and microbiology (including AFB/fungal studies when appropriate).

5.6 Chest drains and closure

Place one basal drain and, in infected or hemothorax cases, an additional apical drain to ensure complete evacuation of air and dependent fluid. Connect to digital suction (-10 to - 20 cmH_2O) initially to quantify air-leak trends; step down to water seal once expansion is satisfactory and the leak is minimal. Port sites are infiltrated with local anesthetic and closed in layers (**Figure 8a–b**). In addition, intercostal nerve blockade or cryoablation can be performed intrathoracically under direct vision before closure to enhance postoperative analgesia (**Figure 9a–b**). The utility incision should accommodate a wound protector to minimize intercostal trauma.

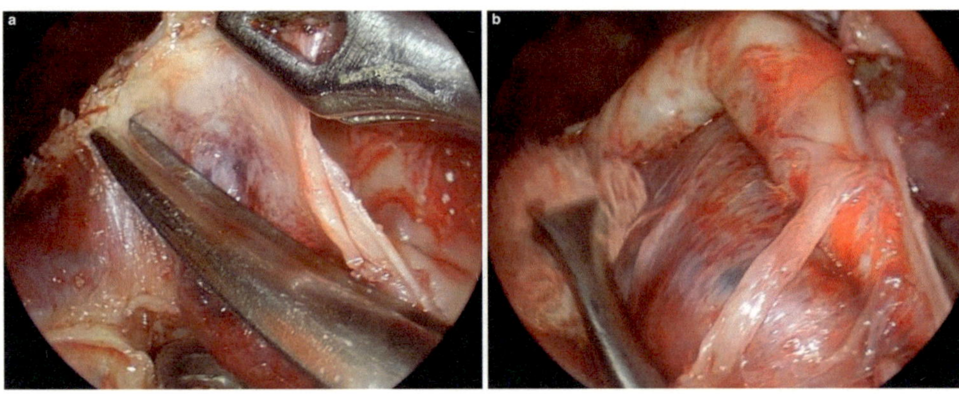

Figure 6.
(a, b). Intraoperative thoracoscopic images illustrating different techniques for visceral peel dissection. (a) Sharp dissection of the plane between the pleural rind and lung parenchyma using scissors. (b) Reverse-direction peeling of the visceral rind while the lung is gently reinflated to facilitate separation.

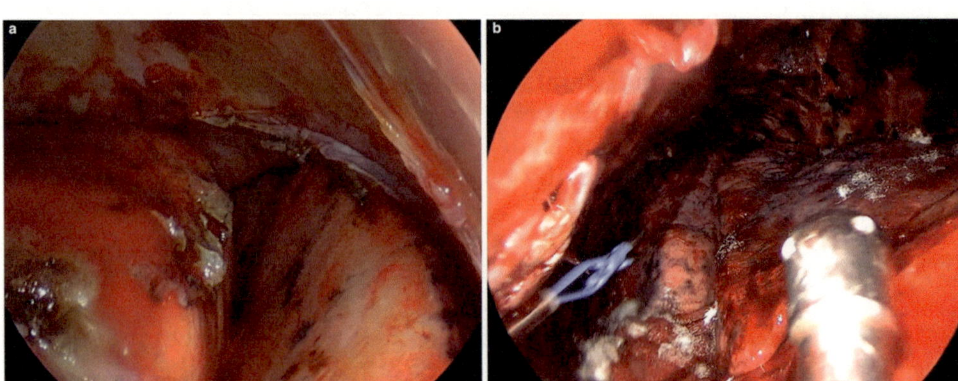

Figure 7.
Post-Decortication Intraoperative View Showing Full Lung Expansion.

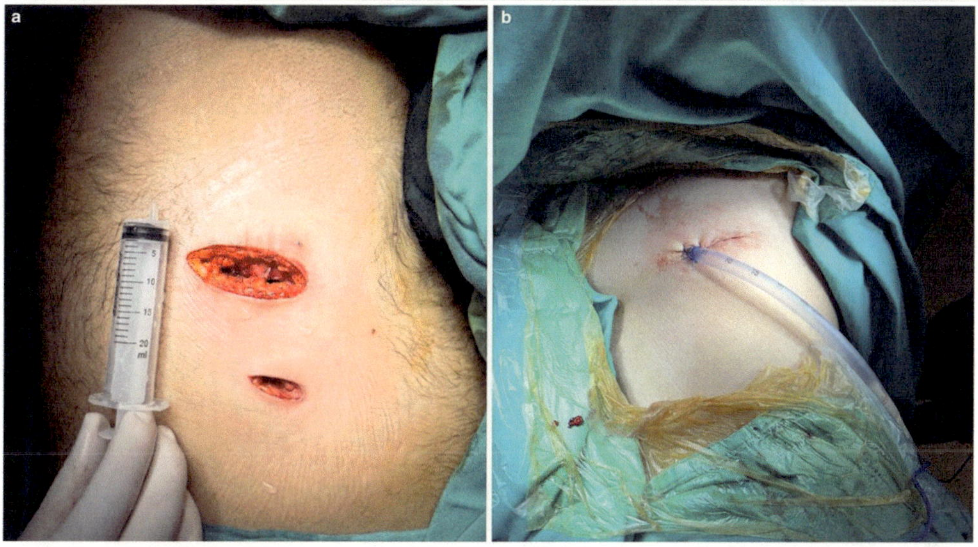

Figure 8.
External View of Port Sites and Uniportal Wound After Decortication.

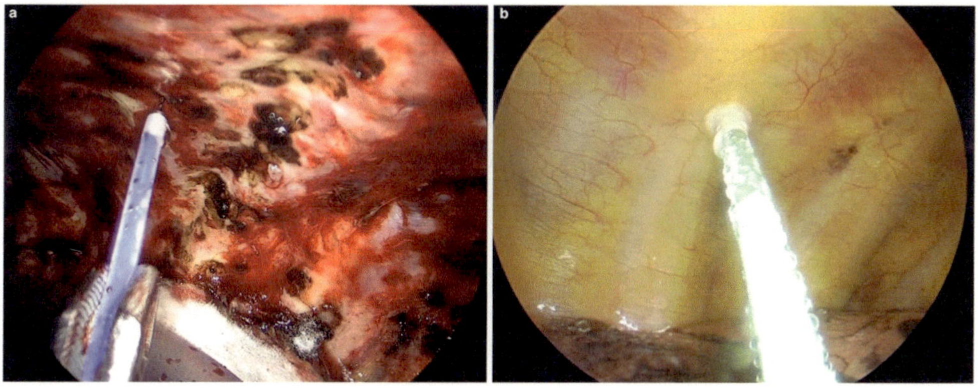

Figure 9.
Thoracoscopic Approach to Intercostal Nerve Block and Cryoablation.

5.7 Conversion thresholds and intraoperative decision-making

Convert early when the plane is unsafe or progress is illusory: diffuse oozing that obscures vision, dense calcified rind with no subpleural glide, uncontrolled bleeding, or failure to achieve near-complete reexpansion after a reasonable period of dissection. Additional triggers include repeated parenchymal tears, deteriorating compliance, or concern for BPF requiring buttressed repair. Establish time and blood-loss guardrails before incision; a calm, planned conversion preserves outcomes and reflects sound judgment.

5.8 Tips, pitfalls, and troubleshooting

Maintain orientation by periodically surveying fixed landmarks (diaphragm, pericardium, fissures). Signs of the wrong plane include bleeding from the lung surface, loss of sheen, and reluctance of segments to expand – stop, reassess, and reenter at a clearer point. Keep instruments long and light in the hand to leverage endoscopic magnification rather than force. When in doubt at the hilum or across obliterated fissures, narrow the dissection corridor and advance in small windows; patience here prevents major air leaks and vascular injury.

6. Special scenarios

6.1 Tuberculous empyema

Tuberculous pleuritis often produces a thick, hypervascular peel with dense fissural adhesions and variable calcification. Expect longer operative times and a higher likelihood of conversion. Antituberculous therapy should be instituted preoperatively whenever feasible and continued postoperatively according to sensitivity testing. Intraoperatively, dissection proceeds with small, sequential "windows" to identify a safe subpleural plane; energy devices are used sparingly on the visceral surface to minimize air-leak risk. Calcified diaphragmatic and mediastinal pleura require deliberate traction–counter-traction with frequent reinflation checks. Bleeding is reduced by keeping the field warm and avoiding unnecessary parietal stripping over intercostal bundles. A low threshold for conversion is appropriate when the plane is obliterated or diffuse oozing compromises visibility [22].

6.2 Postlobectomy/postpneumonectomy space and bronchopleural fistula (BPF)

After lobectomy, persistent space and trapped residual lobes manifest as impaired reexpansion, prolonged drainage, and recurrent infection. VATS decortication can free the visceral rind, allow reexpansion, and, when combined with cavity obliteration (omental or muscle flap in selected cases), eradicate infection. In contrast, chronic postpneumonectomy empyema – especially with BPF – rarely benefits from thoracoscopic decortication alone. Management is staged: control sepsis (drainage and antibiotics), close the fistula (often via an open approach with bronchial stump buttress using muscle or omentum), and obliterate the space (Clagett/modified Clagett, Eloesser window, or muscle transposition) [23]. Thoracoscopy may assist debridement in early, contained cases without fistula, but surgeons should pivot early to an open strategy if contamination is extensive or stump integrity is uncertain [24].

6.3 Retained hemothorax (trauma)

Early VATS (ideally within 48–72 hours) reduces empyema, ventilator days, and ICU length of stay. The aim is to evacuate clots, release septations, and selectively decorticate organized peel to restore expansion. Port placement targets the dependent posterior collections; careful inspection of the diaphragm and lung parenchyma is mandatory to exclude missed injuries. Coagulopathy is corrected preoperatively; intraoperative warming and meticulous hemostasis are essential. Analgesia (paravertebral/ESP block) and aggressive pulmonary physiotherapy accelerate recovery. Delayed presentation with fibrothorax may necessitate more extensive visceral decortication and carries a higher conversion risk [25, 26].

6.4 Pediatric patients

Children have a thinner chest wall, smaller working spaces, and more reactive pleura. Use smaller ports and instruments, limit energy on the visceral surface, and maintain normothermia. Single-lung ventilation may require a bronchial blocker rather than a double-lumen tube in younger patients [25]. Outcomes are excellent when intervention is timely: early VATS drainage and decortication shorten hospital stay, reduce chest-tube days, and minimize the need for thoracotomy. Close collaboration with pediatric anesthesia and physiotherapy teams is pivotal.

6.5 Malignant trapped lung

In malignant pleural disease, decortication is palliative and should be aligned with the goals of care. Candidates are those with symptomatic dyspnea, reasonable performance status, expected survival beyond several months, and focal mechanical restriction rather than diffuse pleural carcinomatosis. Intraoperatively, expect friable pleura and increased bleeding; extensive stripping is avoided if it does not meaningfully improve expansion. If the lung remains nonexpandable, symptom control is achieved with an indwelling pleural catheter (± talc poudrage if partial expansion permits pleurodesis). Multidisciplinary discussions ensure that systemic therapy plans and anticoagulation are coordinated with surgical timing.

Practical summary: these complex scenarios demand a flexible strategy, early recognition of unsafe planes, and readiness to convert or stage the operation. Thoughtful patient selection and close multidisciplinary coordination are the main determinants of success.

7. Outcomes and evidence summary

Across contemporary cohort studies and meta-analyses, VATS has demonstrated superior outcomes compared with open thoracotomy for pleural decortication across multiple clinical parameters. Multiple studies consistently report that VATS offers shorter operative times, reduced postoperative pain, shorter hospital stays, and fewer postoperative complications [27–30]. A meta-analysis of 1,795 patients further confirmed significantly shorter chest tube duration, lower rates of prolonged air leaks, and reduced overall complication rates with VATS [29]. Patients also report higher satisfaction and less surgical trauma [30].

When outcomes are evaluated across modern cohorts, VATS decortication achieves clinical success and lung reexpansion rates comparable to thoracotomy in appropriately selected patients. The minimally invasive approach consistently reduces postoperative pain and opioid consumption, lowers wound morbidity, and shortens hospital stay – without compromising clearance when the subpleural plane is safely developed. Reported conversion rates range from 5% to 30%, mainly reflecting disease chronicity, tuberculous or fungal etiology, pleural calcification, and the patient's physiological reserve rather than a failure of the thoracoscopic technique. Predictors of technical difficulty and conversion include symptom duration beyond 4–6 weeks, a thick or calcified visceral rind, tuberculous empyema, severe malnutrition or immunosuppression, and extensive diaphragmatic or fissural involvement. While early intrapleural enzyme therapy (tPA/DNase) can reduce the need for surgery in the fibrinopurulent phase, once organization is established, VATS decortication remains the definitive method for achieving lung reexpansion and infection control. Open thoracotomy, however, retains a role in complex or densely organized cases requiring extensive decortication.

8. Postoperative management

Postoperative care focuses on infection control, full reexpansion, analgesia, and early mobilization. Antibiotics are culture-directed and typically continued for two to six weeks in empyema, adjusted in concert with infectious diseases teams and clinical response. Analgesia should be multimodal to permit immediate mobilization, incentive spirometry, and chest physiotherapy – measures that reduce atelectasis and expedite discharge.

Physiotherapy and rehabilitation play a central role in postoperative recovery following decortication or VATS. Early respiratory physiotherapy begins within hours after extubation, emphasizing deep-breathing exercises, incentive spirometry, and active coughing to clear secretions and maintain lung reexpansion. Chest wall mobility and shoulder range-of-motion exercises are introduced as soon as pain control allows, preventing stiffness and postthoracotomy syndrome. As the patient stabilizes, ambulation and progressive aerobic activity are encouraged to enhance pulmonary mechanics, improve oxygenation, and reduce the risk of venous thromboembolism.

In patients with prolonged recovery or preexisting pulmonary compromise, structured pulmonary rehabilitation programs – including supervised exercise training, breathing retraining, and patient education – further optimize postoperative function and quality of life. Collaboration between surgeons, physiotherapists, and rehabilitation specialists ensures that each patient follows a personalized recovery plan, balancing safety with early physical engagement.

Chest drain management is guided by objective air leak trends – ideally via digital devices – with stepwise suction weaning and timely removal once the air leak has ceased, drainage is minimal, and radiography confirms near-complete expansion. Anticoagulation is resumed when hemostasis is secure, while venous thromboembolism prophylaxis follows institutional protocols. Nutritional optimization continues postoperatively with early high-protein intake and correction of anemia to support healing and immune function.

9. Complications and management

Persistent air leak is the most frequent issue after decortication and is best mitigated by gentle handling of the visceral pleura and avoidance of excessive suction. Management ranges from continued drainage with physiotherapy to targeted suturing of focal leaks, application of sealants, or selective use of endobronchial valves in prolonged cases. Bleeding demands meticulous intraoperative hemostasis and vigilance in recovery; reexploration is warranted for hemodynamic compromise or ongoing transfusion requirements. Residual collections or persistent pleural space may be addressed with image-guided catheter drainage, a return to the operating room for further decortication, or, in chronic infected cavities, obliteration strategies, including muscle flap transposition. Reexpansion pulmonary edema is uncommon but potentially serious; prevention hinges on gradual evacuation of large chronic spaces, cautious suction settings, and judicious fluid management [31, 32].

10. Learning curve, resources, and adoption

Learning curve, resources, and adoption: successful VATS decortication depends on team experience with minimally invasive thoracic techniques, familiarity with subpleural dissection, and access to appropriate instruments and imaging. Uniportal approaches are feasible once a multiport technique is mastered. Low-volume centers can achieve good outcomes with careful selection, early referral of very chronic or calcified disease, and a low threshold for conversion.

11. Future directions

Robotic platforms are likely to expand the minimally invasive envelope for difficult decortications. Wristed instruments, tremor filtration, and immersive 3-D vision may facilitate fine traction–counter-traction on a tenuous visceral plane, particularly over the fissures and diaphragm, and could reduce the need for wide parietal stripping. Hybrid strategies (VATS access with selective robotic dissection) deserve evaluation in calcified or tuberculous disease, where conversion thresholds are currently low. Adjunctive imaging is another frontier: fluorescence-based perfusion assessment (e.g., indocyanine green) may help judge pleural perfusion and the viability of marginal segments after peel removal, while advanced ultrasound – including shear-wave elastography and micro-Doppler – could map rind thickness and stiffness pre- and intraoperatively to guide port placement and predict plane quality [33, 34].

Digital perioperative analytics should mature from simple thresholds to trend- and risk-based decision support. Objective air-leak curves, drain flow variability, and cough-related spike profiles can be combined with clinical features to standardize drain removal criteria and identify patients at risk of prolonged leak or readmission. Remote monitoring – home spirometry, activity metrics, and patient-reported dyspnea – can be integrated with indwelling catheter/portable drain data to support earlier discharge without compromising safety. Prospective registries with common data elements and linkage to microbiology will enable benchmarking across centers and case-mixes, while machine-learning models may refine selection (e.g., predicting conversion, bleeding risk, or nonexpandable lung) and optimize timing.

Future trials should prioritize pragmatic designs that reflect real-world pathways – adaptive or cluster-randomized comparisons of early VATS versus intrapleural enzyme therapy in stage II disease; stepped-wedge implementations of digital drain protocols; and platform trials evaluating analgesic and rehabilitation bundles. Outcome sets must extend beyond radiographic expansion to include patient-centered measures (dyspnea scores, QoR-15, time to return to normal activity), long-term recurrence/infection control, and cost-effectiveness across different health-system resource levels.

Finally, durable adoption relies on training and implementation science. Proficiency-based curricula using bench models, VR/haptic simulators, and telementoring can shorten the learning curve, while team rehearsals of conversion drills and standardized checklists improve safety. In resource-limited settings, context-adapted instrument sets, reusable device pathways, and simplified digital-drain protocols can broaden access. Collaboration through international registries and consensus processes should clarify indications, technical standards, and reporting terminology so that results are comparable and scalable.

12. Conclusions

VATS decortication has matured into a safe, effective, and durable solution for organized pleural disease when patients are appropriately selected and perioperative care is standardized. Its value derives from three pillars: timely referral based on stage-aware decision-making, meticulous subpleural dissection that restores lung mechanics, and disciplined postoperative pathways that consolidate reexpansion while minimizing complications. In contemporary practice, outcomes – defined by clinical success, reexpansion, and recurrence control – are comparable to thoracotomy but with the advantages of minimal access surgery: less pain, lower wound morbidity, and faster recovery.

Patient selection remains paramount. Cross-sectional imaging and bedside ultrasound should assess peel thickness, calcification, fissural involvement, and the presence of a developable plane; special etiologies such as tuberculous or fungal pleuritis, long symptom duration, and severe malnutrition warrant tempered expectations and a lower threshold for conversion. Conversely, early intervention in retained hemothorax and progressing fibrinopurulent disease improves technical ease and reduces downstream sepsis and fibrothorax. These considerations argue for a pragmatic algorithm that integrates image-guided drainage and intrapleural therapy in early phases with timely VATS once organization is established.

Technical fundamentals are consistent across approaches – multiport or uniportal. Safe progress hinges on precise identification of the subpleural plane, traction–counter-traction rather than energy on the visceral surface, stepwise hemostasis, and periodic reinflation to judge adequacy. Conversion to thoracotomy is a safety maneuver, not a failure; it should occur early when the plane is obliterated, bleeding obscures vision, or full reexpansion cannot be achieved. Postoperatively, culture-directed antibiotics, multimodal analgesia, early mobilization, and objective drain management (preferably digital) underpin reliable recovery.

Complex scenarios require nuance. Postlobectomy space with trapped residual lobes can often be salvaged thoracoscopically; chronic postpneumonectomy empyema with BPF usually mandates staged open strategies and cavity obliteration.

In malignant trapped lung, the role of decortication is palliative and should be aligned with goals of care, with indwelling catheters and selective pleurodesis used to control symptoms when full expansion is unattainable.

Looking forward, incremental gains will likely come from structured training, team rehearsal of conversion protocols, digital drain analytics to standardize removal criteria, and selective adoption of robotic platforms or image-guidance for difficult planes. Prospective registries and pragmatic comparative studies are needed to refine indications, quantify patient-centered outcomes, and define cost-effectiveness across health systems.

In summary, a stage-based, safety-first VATS strategy – supported by thoughtful selection, reproducible technique, and protocolized aftercare – offers the most direct path to lung reexpansion and durable resolution of organized pleural disease.

Author details

Güntuğ Batıhan
Department of Thoracic Surgery, Çanakkale Onsekiz Mart University, Çanakkale, Türkiye

*Address all correspondence to: gbatihan@hotmail.com

References

[1] Rathinam S, Waller DA. Pleurectomy decortication in the treatment of the "trapped lung" in benign and malignant pleural effusions. Thoracic Surgery Clinics. 2013;**23**(1):51–61. DOI: 10.1016/j.thorsurg.2012.10.007

[2] Upadrista PK, Sabbula BR, Akella J. Trapped lung. In: StatPearls [Internet]. Treasure Island (FL): StatPearls Publishing; 2025 Jan-. Available from: https://www.ncbi.nlm.nih.gov/books/NBK564357/ [Accessed: 2023-Feburary-12]

[3] Doelken P. Clinical implications of unexpandable lung due to pleural disease. The American Journal of the Medical Sciences. 2008;**335**(1):21–25. DOI: 10.1097/MAJ.0b013e31815f1a44

[4] Reichert M, Hecker M, Witte B, Bodner J, Padberg W, Weigand MA, Hecker A. Stage-directed therapy of pleural empyema. Langenbeck's Archives of Surgery. 2017;**402**(1):15–26. DOI: 10.1007/s00423-016-1498-9

[5] Bender MT, Ferraris VA, Saha SP. Modern management of thoracic empyema. Southern Medical Journal. 2015;**108**(1):58–62. DOI: 10.14423/SMJ.0000000000000226

[6] Jindal R, Nar AS, Mishra A, Singh RP, Aggarwal A, Bansal N. Video-assisted thoracoscopic surgery versus open thoracotomy in the management of empyema: A comparative study. Journal of Minimal Access Surgery. 2021;**17**(4):470–478. DOI: 10.4103/jmas.JMAS_249_19

[7] Godfrey MS, Bramley KT, Detterbeck F. Medical and surgical management of empyema. Seminars in Respiratory and Critical Care Medicine. 2019;**40**(3):361–374. DOI: 10.1055/s-0039-1694699

[8] Steen K, Sørensen J, Christensen M, Petersen RH, Naidu B, Bendixen M, Rahman NM, Laursen CB, Christensen TD. Comparison of video assisted thoracoscopic surgery and thoracotomy for treatment of pleural infection stage II and III: A literature review. Journal of Thoracic Disease. 2023;**15**(11):6323–6332. DOI: 10.21037/jtd-23-928

[9] Reichert M, Pösentrup B, Hecker A, Padberg W, Bodner J. Lung decortication in phase III pleural empyema by video-assisted thoracoscopic surgery (VATS)-results of a learning curve study. Journal of Thoracic Disease. 2018;**10**(7):4311–4320. DOI: 10.21037/jtd.2018.06.72

[10] McCauley L, Dean N. Pneumonia and empyema: Causal, casual or unknown. Journal of Thoracic Disease. 2015;7(6):992–998. DOI: 10.3978/j.issn.2072-1439.2015.04.36

[11] Sorino C, Mondoni M, Lococo F, Marchetti G, Feller-Kopman D. Optimizing the management of complicated pleural effusion: From intrapleural agents to surgery. Respiratory Medicine. 2022;**191**:106706. DOI: 10.1016/j.rmed.2021.106706

[12] De Vera CJ, Emerine RL, Girard RA, Sarva K, Jacob J, Azghani AO, Florence JM, Cook A, Norwood S, Singh KP, Komissarov AA, Florova G, Idell S. A novel rabbit model of retained hemothorax with pleural organization. International Journal of Molecular Sciences. 2023;**25**(1):470. DOI: 10.3390/ijms25010470

[13] Weissberg D, Refaely Y. Pleural empyema: 24-year experience. The Annals of Thoracic Surgery. 1996;**62** (4):1026–1029. DOI: 10.1016/0003-4975(96)00494-8

[14] Zhou Y, Li X, Dai J, Lin L, Cao X, Liu X, Jiang G. Uniportal thoracoscopic decortication for stage III tuberculous empyema with severe rib crowding. The Annals of Thoracic Surgery. 2021;**112** (1):289–294. DOI: 10.1016/j.athoracsur.2020.07.067

[15] Ravaglia C, Gurioli C, Tomassetti S, Casoni GL, Romagnoli M, Gurioli C, Agnoletti V, Poletti V. Is medical thoracoscopy efficient in the management of multiloculated and organized thoracic empyema? Respiration. 2012;**84**(3):219–224. DOI: 10.1159/000339414

[16] Rusch VW. Pleurectomy and decortication: How I teach it. The Annals of Thoracic Surgery. 2017;**103** (5):1374–1377. DOI: 10.1016/j.athoracsur.2017.02.042

[17] Pulle MV, Asaf BB, Kumar A, Puri HV, Vijay CL, Bishnoi S. Microbiological profile of tubercular and nontubercular empyemas and its impact on clinical outcomes: A retrospective analysis of 285 consecutively operated cases. Lung India. 2020;**37**(5):389–393. DOI: 10.4103/lungindia.lungindia_553_19

[18] Agostini P, Singh S. Incentive spirometry following thoracic surgery: What should we be doing? Physiotherapy. 2009;**95**(2):76–82. DOI: 10.1016/j.physio.2008.11.003

[19] Chen B, Zhang J, Ye Z, Ye M, Ma D, Wang C, Zhu C. Outcomes of video-assisted thoracic surgical decortication in 274 patients with tuberculous empyema. Annals of Thoracic and Cardiovascular Surgery. 2015;**21**(3):223–228. DOI: 10.5761/atcs.oa.14-00185

[20] Rahman NM, Maskell NA, Davies CW, Hedley EL, Nunn AJ, Gleeson FV, Davies RJ. The relationship between chest tube size and clinical outcome in pleural infection. Chest. 2010;**137**(3):536–543. DOI: 10.1378/chest.09-1044

[21] Corcoran JP, Psallidas I, Gerry S, Piccolo F, Koegelenberg CF, Saba T, Daneshvar C, Fairbairn I, Heinink R, West A, Stanton AE, Holme J, Kastelik JA, Steer H, Downer NJ, Haris M, Baker EH, Everett CF, Pepperell J, Bewick T, Yarmus L, Maldonado F, Khan B, Hart-Thomas A, Hands G, Warwick G, De Fonseka D, Hassan M, Munavvar M, Guhan A, Shahidi M, Pogson Z, Dowson L, Popowicz ND, Saba J, Ward NR, Hallifax RJ, Dobson M, Shaw R, Hedley EL, Sabia A, Robinson B, Collins GS, Davies HE, Yu LM, Miller RF, Maskell NA, Rahman NM. Prospective validation of the RAPID clinical risk prediction score in adult patients with pleural infection: The PILOT study. European Respiratory Journal. 2020; **56** (5):2000130. DOI: 10.1183/13993003.00130-2020

[22] Huang CL, Zhang W, Ni ZY, Zuo T, Zhou M, Xu J, Yang ZF, Li L, Xiao J, Zhang DY. Efficacy of video-assisted thoracoscopic surgery for 29 patients with tuberculosis-destroyed lung. International Journal of Clinical and Experimental Medicine. 2015;**8** (10):18391–18398

[23] Miller Jr JI. The history of surgery of empyema, thoracoplasty, Eloesser flap, and muscle flap transposition.

Chest Surgery Clinics of North America. 2000;**10**(1):45–53

[24] Torigoe H, Toyooka S, Yamamoto H, Soh J, Miyoshi S. Usefulness of thoracoscopic debridement for chronic empyema after an extrapleural pneumonectomy. Acta Medica Okayama. 2016;**70**(6):507–510. DOI: 10.18926/AMO/54816

[25] Smith JW, Franklin GA, Harbrecht BG, Richardson JD. Early VATS for blunt chest trauma: A management technique underutilized by acute care surgeons. The Journal of Trauma. 2011;**71**(1):102–107. DOI: 10.1097/TA.0b013e3182223080

[26] Lin HL, Huang WY, Yang C, Chou SM, Chiang HI, Kuo LC, Lin TY, Chou YP. How early should VATS be performed for retained haemothorax in blunt chest trauma? Injury. 2014;**45** (9):1359–1364. DOI: 10.1016/j.injury.2014.05.036

[27] Tong BC, Hanna J, Toloza EM, Onaitis MW, D'Amico TA, Harpole DH, Burfeind WR. Outcomes of video-assisted thoracoscopic decortication. The Annals of Thoracic Surgery. 2010;**89**(1):220–225. DOI: 10.1016/j.athoracsur.2009.09.021

[28] Elbasiouny ARM, ElNory AA, Mostafa AM, ElDewer MA. Video-assisted thoracoscopic decortication versus open decortication for better surgical results. The Egyptian Journal of Surgery. 2024;**43**(4):1463–1470. DOI: 10.21608/EJSUR.2024.293633.1090

[29] Sudarma IW, Yasa KP, Harta IKAP, Pertiwi PFK. Video-assisted thoracoscopic surgery vs. open thoracotomy in the management of empyema: A meta-analytical perspective. Journal of Innovation in Medical and Applied Sciences (JINAVA). 2024;**4**(2). DOI: 10.51559/jinava.v4i2.72

[30] Chan DTL, Sihoe ADL, Chan S, Tsang DSF, Fang B, Lee TW, Cheng LC. Surgical treatment for empyema thoracis: Is video-assisted thoracic surgery "better" than thoracotomy? Annals of Thoracic Surgery. 2007;**84** (1):225–231. DOI: 10.1016/j.athoracsur.2007.03.019

[31] Venuta F, Rendina EA, De Giacomo T, Coloni GF. Postoperative strategies to treat permanent air leaks. Thoracic Surgery Clinics. 2010;**20**(3):391–397. DOI: 10.1016/j.thorsurg.2010.03.004

[32] Hashimoto M, Kondo N, Nakamichi T, Nakamura A, Kuroda A, Takuwa T, Matsumoto S, Hasegawa S. Control of air leakage during pleurectomy/decortication by the ventilation and anchoring method. General Thoracic and Cardiovascular Surgery. 2022;**70**(8):730–734. DOI: 10.1007/s11748-022-01789-4

[33] Tung KH, Yendamuri S, Seastedt KP. Adoption of the robotic platform across thoracic surgeries. Journal of Clinical Medicine. 2024;**13** (19):5764. DOI: 10.3390/jcm13195764

[34] Siu ICH, Li Z, Ng CSH. Latest technology in minimally invasive thoracic surgery. Annals of Translational Medicine. 2019;**7**(2):35. DOI: 10.21037/atm.2018.12.47